The Family who play together have More Fun!

But, to me, it currently is a situation in the vast majority of households that the following applies:-

The family
who <u>played</u>
together
<u>had</u> more fun!

AND IS THAT NOW AN ANOCHRONISTIC [1] *RETROSPECTIVE REALITY?*

1 = Something belonging or appropriate to an earlier period, especially so as to seem conspicuously old-fashioned or outdated.

I suppose here I should start by saying that this Book is directed at those get together families who actually play together indoors AND outdoors – or where the kids plus friends venture into the garden and play competitively - where the I-Pad has not become the main post pram child distractor – where the mention of the great outdoors has become taboo as the great indoors seat in front of an immobile screen have become the new exercise regime machinery – where 'getting out of breath' has become an anachronistic [1] term, replaced by repetitive finger/thumb strain injuries!!!

AND in so many households the parents/children become detached physically as well as, dare I say, emotionally!

AND from this situation there emanates the loss of the inter child/parent connectivity:- that bond seems to have slowly began to disappear!

AND dare I say its replacement is not one that could have been easily perceived by those taking the easy parenting way out, well possibly not, with those who openly encouraged the split?

BUT the contrary argument could be that in the pre mass produced computer technologically based inter active games days, there was always that parent/child split:- where the child had <u>free outside</u> rein!

AND in those days they could easily, as all their neighbouring friends would be out there also:- the girl/boy standard games would be such like, the well known skipping, hopscotch, football &/or cricket, or use of marbles &/or collector cards, or that now outlawed conker battles!

BUT there were plenty about my patient John related to me which would be a little too physical for the now overprotective mothers, as well as they took place in the streets, whose roadway now totally belongs to the might automobile, which might also be described as the silent (electric powered?) killer!

When Grandad/Ma were young, those post war days:

It was Rough'nTough - Not Like Today!

<u>We had to make our own fun!</u> – <u>We had to improvise!</u>

Even if what we did at times resembled Battle Encounters!

Those bygone days, before the Current Health & Safety Executives existed, we had NoBody looking out for EveryThing & EveryOne!

So, what we got up to on the streets **<u>AND</u>** at school would now give them a Severe Pulmonary! (And, if condoned, the sack?)

So, let's see if you Modern Mums & Dads would agree?

The first thing you should appreciate, those days the streets were our unsupervised playground and the one in our school(s) were a case of survival of/by the ????

So, get ready for some good old Tears / Black Eyes / Bruising / Bumping / Bleeding Hands & Knees, ***Fifties-Sixties*** Style!!!

1. **<u>Ball Toss</u>** then would have a different connotation, to this day: there we would not be thrown to, rather thrown at, as we all lined up against the Wire Fencing trying valiantly to avoid being hit by the many tennis balls being thrown our way – be hit and you're out. Many's a time the way to avoid being struck-out (pardon the Americanism Non-Link) was to run behind some unsuspecting one, or failing this, just yank them in front of you!
2. **<u>Bulldog</u>** had no canine link! Here it was the word used as the catcher(s) lifted their opponent off the ground and claimed him/her as one of their own and he/she then helped them grab more of the opposition who tried to run past them to the Home Base (again sorry for the Americanism Non-Link), then tried to run back.
3. **<u>Chain Gang</u>** had neither gang nor chain links (sorry for the inexcusable pun)! Here the joined arms were the body parts which you struggled to avoid getting yours! Like No2 it was a case of running from one side of the playground without being caught.
   a. The original catchers would be formed of 2 reasonably good runners, standing side-to-side with one pair of hands joined together, which link they were not allowed to break, thus extending their reach.
   b. They would try to wrap their extended arms about someone running their way, thus increasing their Human Chain to three.
   c. Then, in true Quiddler fashion (below) if the three caught another, making 4: these 4 would then split into two pairs,

and so on, until all were caught, or the end of playtime whistle was blown!

    d. The most common injury was the runner's avoiding capture ending up having his/her head being chopped off! No, silly, but head high *tackles* were quite common; + one of the chain members in a threesome having both their arms metaphorically ripped off by the runner to their left & right going in opposite directions! And the occasional trip, as the Chain member tried to obstruct the runner! Oh I mustn't also forget the regular face high, wrestling type fore hand smash! Oh and the usual collisions, unintentionally running into each other, here and there avoiding being caught!

4. <u>**The Ball Gang**</u> Very similar to No3, but with a possible painful ending guaranteed – depending how unpopular you were with the throwers ganging up on you!

    a. Again you start off with two, here throwing the ball at people and if they hit any then they join their Ball Gang trying to hit others, but it was not all loaded in the thrower's favour.

    b. None of the gang were allowed to run with the ball, (A sort of stationary Lacrosse!) they had to rely on the other gang members to run into an advantageous position to hit someone with the ball if they had it: hence the person with the ball being aware where his Gang partners were situated and throw it to the best positioned before the object runner was out of range.

c. So, if a Ball gang member were right on top of you and in possession of the ball it would be painful curtains out for you? Actually no, as the person trying to be hit had one piece in his armoury, that of hand defence: so if he were to deflect the ball with his hand it would not count as he being caught. He could then run away and be tried to be re-caught, so to speak. Not always a sensible tactic↓!

d. Well, injuries were like above, but additionally charging inadvertently into some innocent in the playground not playing your game (Yes we played this at break-time!) as we dodged flying balls; getting one in the back/legs/face which hurt because the Ball Gang Member was right on top of you when he hurled the ball as hard as he could ↑at you: here it paid to be popular, those not, got bruised far more often!

e. One final self-preservation rule in this Boys Only School: Never be face-on to a ball throwing Gang Member, or, put into Common Cockney Anglo Saxon parlance, don't put your crown jewels head-on target practice display – get me? I know one who did and he wasn't a happy *male* bunny for several days afterwards!

f. Other than that serious injury the usual casualties were yanked tie, ripped shirts and a torn jacket here & there!

5. **<u>The Tunnel Run</u>** This the least dangerous game which <u>**you**</u> might try playing in an *limited* open space – I say limited because if it is too large it will spoil part of the under arm throwing element of the game, if all ages are involved!

   a. I actually forgot the original name, but you'll get my *tunnel* drift later on. This is educational on a certain level, as the young-uns would learn from the old-uns: the age range being 6-10, then. But, there is no reason all ages cannot join in.

   b. Say you start with 6 kids, one is the first ball-tosser (BT) and he/she is asked to go away from the remainder of the group, after he/she has given the rest the category for their round. Say it was fruit. The 5 would agree a fruit name for each of them and most importantly, one for the (BT).

   c. When ready, the (BT) is recalled to the group and one of the 5 then recites the 6 fruit names to him/her.

   d. The (BT) then decides which he thinks was not ascribed to him/her and calls out that name, as the ball is tossed <u>vertically</u> above them all.

   e. Now as he/she begins the toss and name call, the other 5 can either run away as far/fast as they can, or delay and hope the (BT) calls his/her own fruit name.

   f. If (BT) calls their own name they lose a life (Everybody starts with just 3 each!), But, and this is the Big

Scampering But, if (BT) calls someone else's fruit name then two things can happen >

g. If the person whose name was called catches the ball, then (BT) loses a life and he/she become (BT) for another round.

h. BUT if person does not and it bounces, then he/she must retrieve it as soon as possible and then scream out Stop – <u>all must obey</u> – those who do not must go back to where they should have been when Stop was called out! (So no cheating!)

i. Now the Ball Holder looks around to see the person nearest to attack! He/she has 3 long strides and 6 pigeon [NB] toe steps to get near to their prey, so to speak. [NB] *Nothing really to do with the medical Term, Intoeing, but here, pointed in the same direction, just placing one foot directly in front of the other ie alternate heel to toe/heel to toe etc.*

j. The Ball Holder must then hit the person with an underarm throw: the person must not move their feet from the ground, but can wiggle/gesticulate as much as they wish to put the thrower off.

k. If the person is hit they lose a life and become (BT) for the next round.

l. If the Ball Holder misses, then they lose a life and become (BT) for the next round, where they choose the subject matter etc...!

m. But, I should admit that there was a certain bending of our local rules by those determined not to lose. One example would be that they did run ups for each of their long stride: rather like the triple jump rather than standing jump!

n. Why was not losing 3 lives so important? Well the self-same people were out to be part of the Tunnel AND NOT the Run.

o. The person to lose 3 lives was to tunnel-run the gauntlet, a beating by the rest and this is how it went >

p. The 5 would line up aside a wall (a couple of feet, or more than half a metre - between individuals); the left hand resting shoulder high against the wall, the right hand ready to do its damage to the tunnel-runner.

q. When all lined up there was a tunnel-gap to run through: run as fast as you can to avoid the many bottom slaps &/or punches by the rest!

r. (With the occasional knee trying to hinder your progress!)

s. (Although your knee in that/their obstructing leg usually put paid to that tactic!)

t. (And worse still, **a dead leg** if their outer leg, with exposed upper thigh part, was *accurately* kneed into whilst trying to block you!)

u. See I said it wasn't so bad!

BUT, those 'invented' game days cost virtually nothing to enjoy!?

AND so back to nowadays with a simple introduction to what the first part of the Book is about:- ***Those in the USA and now most other Countries us the meal takeaway facilities offered on-line etc > the humble pizza.***
BUT, and it is my Standard Big But, why throw away the box it was contained in?
BUT >>>

BE CAREFUL OF PIZZAS THEY CAN BITE BACK!

If you were to view 'Pinterest' under cardboard crocodiles you'd get masses of images, but, notwithstanding all that imagery put on view before you, the one I have in mind is not there.
And so we don't even have to go down the 'Amazon' route ## as the humble used Pizza Box has all the Crocodile you'll need!
Well you might? >>> ***What is silly about it all** is that you can buy unmade pizza box es on-line for less than the cost of a Pizza and yet get it delivered to your door in an even greater cardboard box you can use later for another project ## courtesy of 'Amazon'!*

Anyhow >>>

Now the food has been eaten and the box dried off you can attack it with your scissors: alternatively set the kids a challenge.

<> *Here it is best they have a used box of their own with the sole proviso it will fit over their individual head!*

Cut a set of smaller teeth into the front flaps into the front opening ends; cut a set of larger teeth into the side opening ends. **(See Below)** Now you have the teeth sorted, it is time for the head: it is important that the oval hollow you cut into the base allows your youngster to poke his/her head through such that their eyes are showing when you open the Pizza Box Biter Surprise. The simple expedient is cut the hole such that the box drops below the eye line but no further as the protruding ears/nose prevent this! The top hole is smaller on purpose so that the top of the head does not fall over the child's eyes etc!

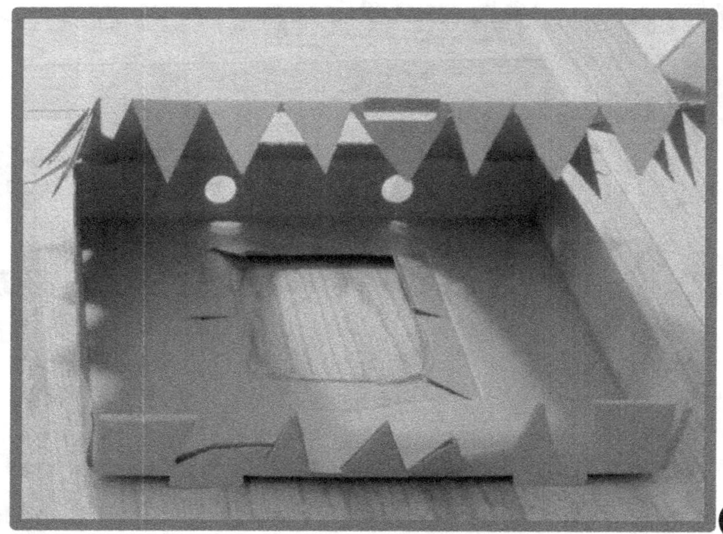**(From Above):-**

There are holes in the top as well as the bottom on purpose: this is so I can fold the top over the child's head and then secure it in place to the lower part with sticky tape so it doesn't flop off!

One piece of advice: you will find the lower front flap is made up of two pieces which fold over and click into grooves to secure them - you should therefore be very careful cutting this lower set of teeth so you don't cut the area where the grooves are as you'll find your teeth flopping over. I actually cut this area for the kids as the extra thickness of the fold is too tough for them to cut without painful pressure on their fingers. *(But there is an alternative – see below)* ***.

↑ Note that the left/right edge end bits need tidying up & it keeps the front ↑ stable/rigid – the above is a poorly cut front example.

There again you find it simpler/easier to cut the front fold in half and not worry about fitting into the grooves? It's all up/down to you out there!
But, perhaps, unnecessary? ***

Once the head is perfected then if you have girls who like to dress up you can then add the elaborate clothing to offset the evil looking head!

But, if you have boisterous boys then the area below the neck can decked over with those trusted, used cardboard box(es): you can add the armour *'plating'* to both sides of the body, kept in place with string over the shoulders and around the tummy areas. ##

Then comes the trusty cardboard cut-out shield, sword and a new helmet if/when the crocodile head is not wanted in their 'new' own warrior scenario!

Here are some attempt(er)s below (Just a Six Year Old) ↓↓↓

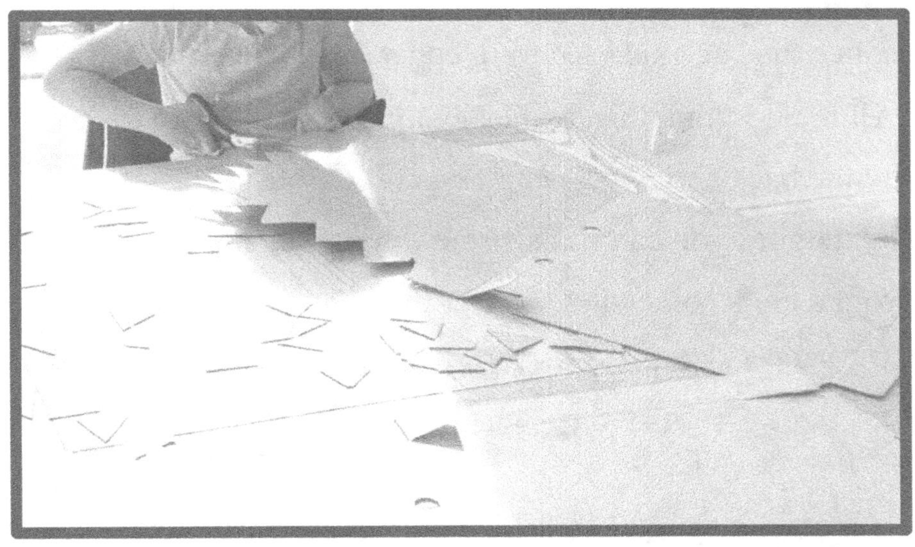

*** *You don't need to fold in the front lap: let it hang loose; you can than*

forget about the side securing edge inserts, just cut them off completely.

The front lower teeth will protrude more, so perhaps that's a good thing

from the picture beneath >>>

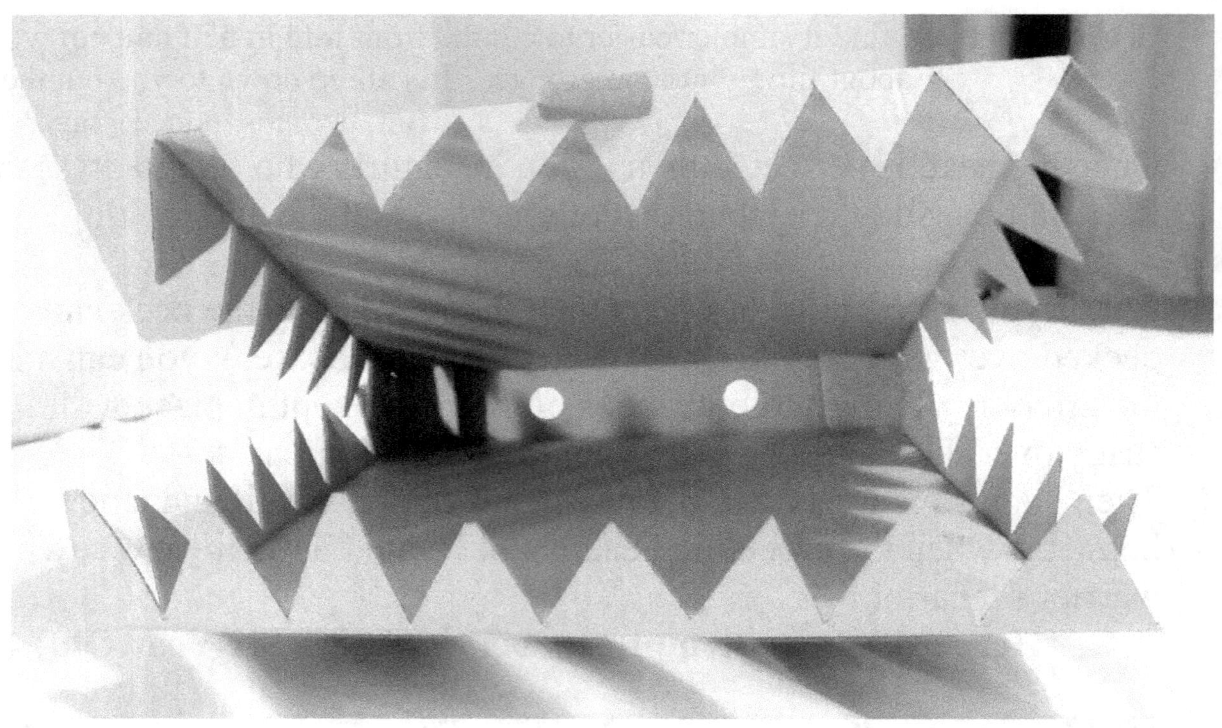

As you will notice the back side securing edges have been retained.

All in all I think this the best cutting plan?

Pity the back eerie holes can't be at the front?

Although as adapting goes you can run a string through them and use it to hang the head from a hook somewhere, rather than have it lying around?

NB THE HOLES E.G. FOR THE HEAD, TOP & BOTTOM HAVE YET TO BE CUT.

OFF YOU GO TRY ME <> Bye for now?

So, effectively that cost you nothing, as opposed to that which modern technology provides at, some say, an exorbitant cost as each year something new comes on the market even more costly than its predecessor – Apple stuff an example where the new model doesn't work with the old connector/piece – if you get my drift?

AND SO I-PADS + GAMES
COST SO MUCH
HERE IDEAS ON A SHOESTRING FOR
THOSE NOT SO WELL OFF!?
OR STRIVE FOR SOMETHING MORE
ENGAGING AND CHALLENGING!?

THINGS FOR
ALL SEASONS
AND EVENTS
BEGINNING WITH
PRE-CHRISTMAS
OCTOBER/NOVEMBER TIMES

<u>NB</u>: *Any item below tagged as (I = indoor) (O = outdoor activity) (I/O = Both)*
(B = Birthdays) (HSG = Home/Social Gatherings)(X = Xmas)

AND so now another preview of what is to come:-
The *'people get ready'* notification that their Christmas
Celebration is coming, for so many, is triggered/announced by
their own Big Bang Halloween/Guy Fawkes celebrations,
which will lead into the following...?!

THAT PRE-CHRISTMAS CAKE MAKING (PT 1) *(X/ I)*

Here we have the standard family get together where the Halloween lit up Pumpkin Face + doorstep trick-or-treat take evening centre stage.

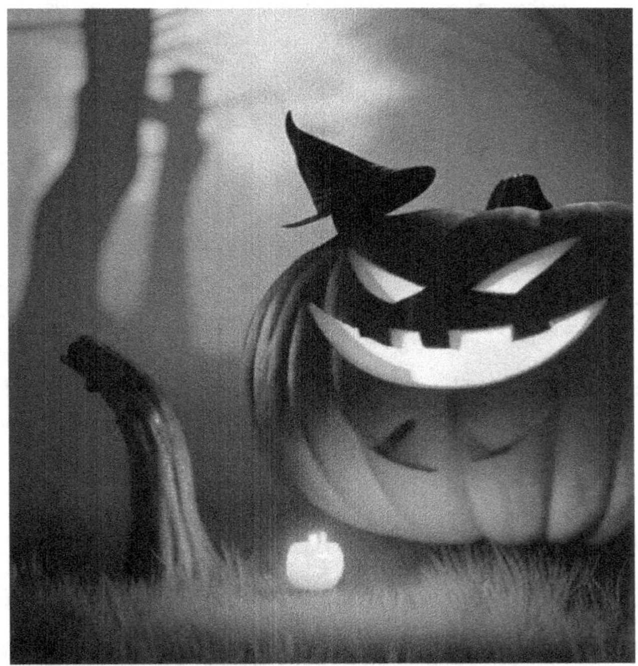

Many pixabay thanks to Roses_Street generated-7523749_1280

Then a week later that annual staged bonfire + firework display!

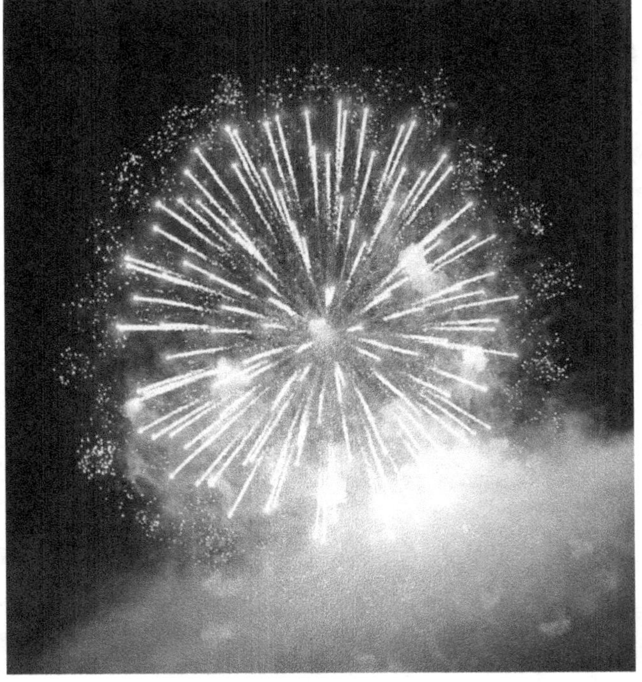

Many pixabay thanks to GregSabin fireworks-6192517_1280

BUT within certain interactive kitchen sharing households, the first part of Christmas Inter-Activity begins at the same time:- it is none other than that 'two-part' Christmas Cake making/baking/covering!

NB **The full cake** making/baking/covering is contained much later in this Book … although Christmas Fun comes early/earlier here a few pages hence where the children's Xmas morning present opening is orchestrated from their parents enjoying more warm bed time! Confused?

All will become much clearer when you read my shortly to appear *CHRISTMAS MORNING WITH AN ENERGETIC DIFFERENCE*!

However [1], here I will include certain aspects to show the 'fun' side of a mother/child/children mix, in the baking/preparation arena.

However [2], here I will point out that you should expect one or two calamities along the way.

And a kitchen holds so much..to go wrong!
As Mummy remembers calamitous/disastrous messes of the past!

"Be careful taking the eggs out of the fridge!"
"Whoops!"

Too late – CRASH!   And so the mess could begin? Like this?

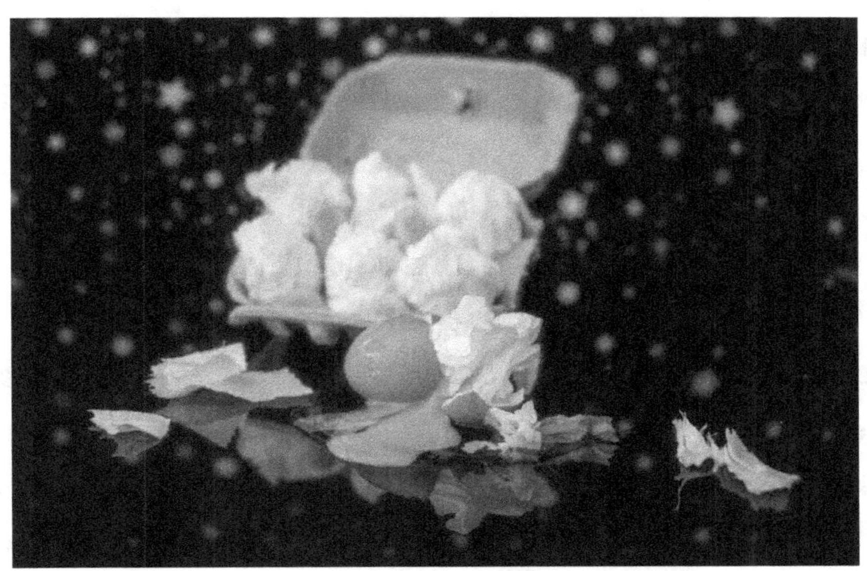

Many thanks to pexels-magda-ehlers-pexels-4097189

>>>>>>>>>>>>>

"Be careful taking the plate out of the cupboard!"
"Whoops!"
Too late – CRASH Number 1!
And so the mess could begin?

Like this?

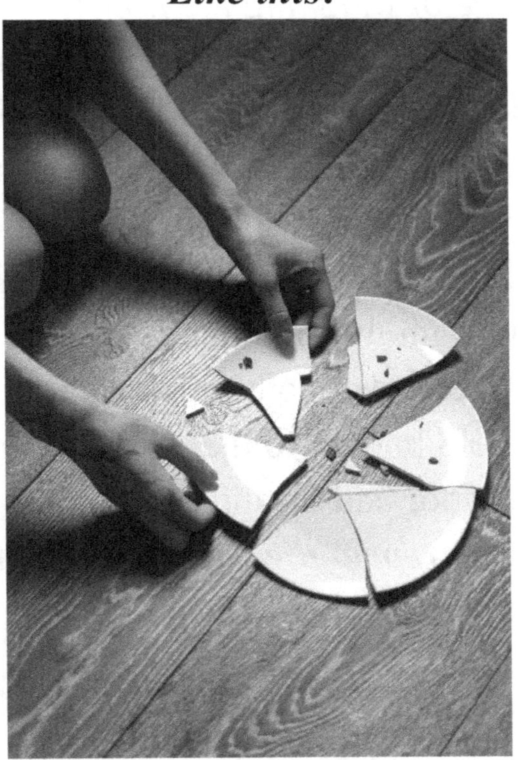

Many thanks to pexels-cottonbro-6717616

So, in that shown directly above, the word of caution/warning, where possible use plastic plates!

AND here I will skip a few stages to re-show the areas of mishap concern!

- Then out came the soaked fruit, for later.
- Next came the weighing of ingredients by each in turn;
- The 200g (8oz) glace cherries in its plastic container.
- ***"Jack take them out one by one, cut each into 2 halves then leave them on the plate next to you and when finished, wash & dry your hands. Then wait for Jill to do her bit."***
- ***Well needless to say Jack found the job a little too sticky for his feeble efforts, as so much of the yucky sticky, gooey mess went onto his hands then his apron!*** *('Thank goodness for the apron!' Mummy whispered to herself.)*
- Jill was in charge of the weighing machine prepared by Mummy.
- But here Mummy knew the mess might start...
- *Jill was in charge of weighing the flour*!
- First came the 6oz plain flour and pouring the right amount out proved a problem as the excess spray flew around all sides of the weighing scale bowl into which all was supposed to go into.
- Needless to say she poured far too much on her first try.
- So it was a case of brushing off the excess on the sides, back into the packet (With the anticipated overspill onto the floor) – Mummy knew there were to be such calamities and had the charged, hand held hoover to the ready – **whoosh/whoosh** and the flour on the floor had disappeared up the hoover spout!
- *RP* ***Get the child to repeat the words the hoover made*** **whoosh/whoosh** *as he/she will soon be asked to repeat them, again/again...*
- The excess flour in the bowl was sorted by Mummy giving Jill a table spoon to scoop it up and put it back into its original packet.

➢ <u>Now Jill knew what not to do</u>, she continued using the spoon to take out the self-raising flour and slowly pouring it on top of the plain flour until the magical 9oz marker came up.

➢ <u>Now came a more difficult job</u> – it looks easy below ↓

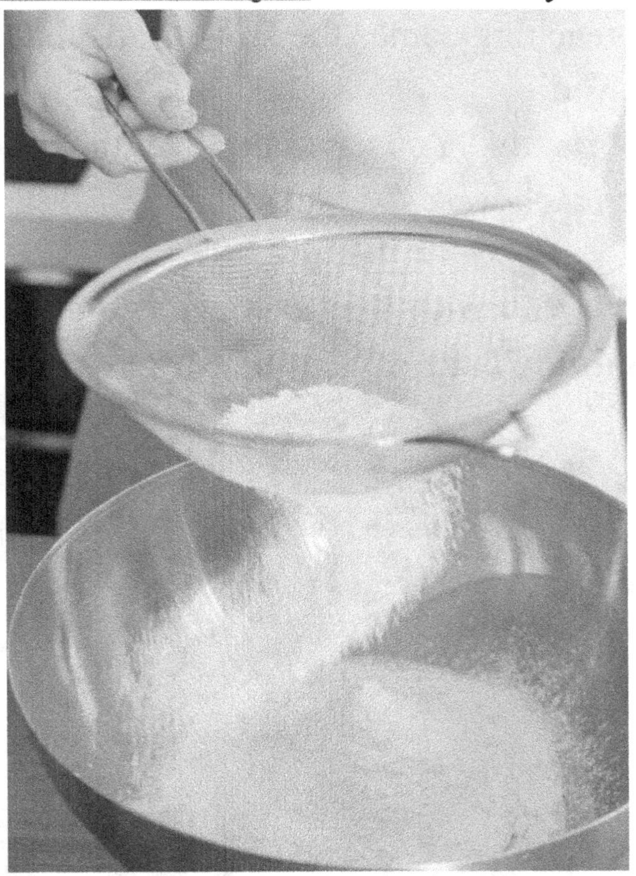

the bake flour sift Many thanks to pexels-meruyert-gonullu-8290267

<u>*(It looks easy – BUT it isn't as Jill would testify!)*</u>

AND the last pre-washing up stage would be the excess cake mix licking up:- and here I might meet objection/criticism as the cake mix would have included the alcohol well-soaked fruit?

Well in this over <u>*'mollycoddled'*</u> era, I'd just say "You're being plain silly, as the alcohol content consumed would be extremely minimal and the whole point is to show how well rewarded some jobs helping Mummy can be!

AND the reward factor plays a significant part in so much of what is to follow.

BUT it will be no 'winner takes all' path we will take, as losers get
their taking part reward also! *

AND for me competitiveness is something to be encouraged, rather
than this cry and get all without effort modern 'child' regime.

BUT with such teaching comes the hometruths that there are rules to
be followed/obeyed.

AND more importantly "You cannot win all the time!"

*Although I have this covered! ***

**AND here I leave you with that unforgettable messy face of joy
where the remaining cake mix is there to be tummy-fully enjoyed!**

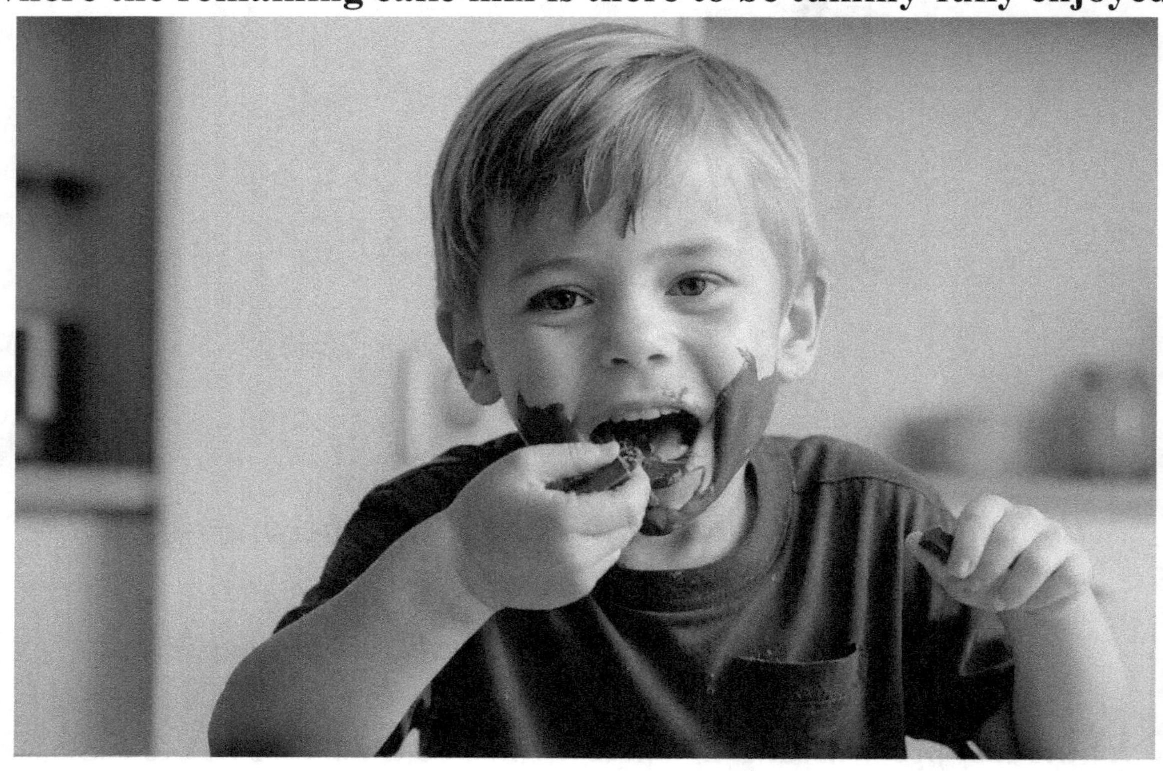

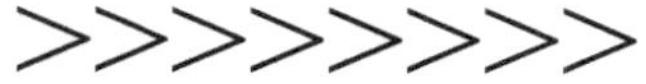

>>>>>>>>>

(Here we will leave this domestic scene – the post bake stage will
make its appearance at the end of the Book, highlighting the
second reward for helping Mummy stage, as jam/marzipan/icing
sugar take their individual (eat me) centre stages!

MY COMPLETE CAKE MAKING PROCESS COMES LATER

>>>>>>>>>

AND HERE NOW ARRIVES MY >>>

CHRISTMAS MORNING WITH AN ENERGETIC DIFFERENCE!

AND here, as parents, join me in my cosy 8am warm bed:-

For the first of my unique present opening games >>>>>

Here the staircase, if you have one, will greatly add to the excited screams of joy environment –

IT IS GREAT TO HEAR HAPPY KIDS!

AND HERE IS MY CHILDHOOD HOME CHRISTMAS MORNING HELTER SKELTER EXPERIENCE!

(Mya) **'I did this with my children, as did my children with theirs!'**

Every Parents Xmas Easy Does It Morning

Tell the kids not to get up until the clock alarm sounds: (Set it for a reasonable time like 8am) - this can give you more controlled sleep.

When it sounds they come to your bedroom and you hand each their Father Christmas Bag(s) with instructions that they may not open any present until the final clue says it is OK!

Then, hand the first clue to the elder (better reader) ~ (No reader see below) where their _first_ present and next clue are situated (usually at the top of the house) (the next at the bottom and so forth – you'll love the excited staircase ** scampering up & down and screeches as they find each present – it's such a wonderful sound, kids enjoying themselves to the full!

Then they'll get to say (?) number 5, the last, with instructions to return with their now full bag(s) to their room & not to open until the last present is found there!

Co-incidentally this final present and a bag to place all the discarded wrappings would be found back in their own room, say, under their respective beds.

The parental pleasure felt as the kids rush, bounding up & down, around the home, with gleeful noises abounding, is such a great feeling!

↑ ~ Obviously if the child/children cannot read they need come to you as they find each present.

Word of caution _make the present easy to find and **easier** to open,_ by your little _Xmas Searchers_, otherwise you'll be dragged out of your warm, comfortable, Xmas snuggle/cuddle up bed.

....

** _The stairway/staircase plays it part in many other indoor games_ ↓

And

Now onto warmer outdoor climes where frsh air contact is made:-

Inventive

'household'

games

for all

playful

Age(d)

groups!

<u>**PART 1:-**</u>
<u>**NB:**</u> *Any item below tagged as (I = indoor) (O = outdoor activity) (I/O = Both)*
(B = Birthdays) (HSG = Home/Social Gatherings)(X = Xmas)

1st.	*HOUSEHOLD PLAYTHINGS*	*I/O*
2nd.	*YOUR PLAYLIST*	*I/O*
3rd.	*POST WARTIME ROUGH & TUMBLES*	*O*
4th.	*HERE THE 'A1' FUN FINALLY BEGINS*	*I/O*
5th.	*KNOCK 'EM OVER*	*I/O*
6th.	*MAKE A WINNING SPLASH*	*O*
7th.	*MAKE A FOOTBALL SPLASH*	*O*
8th.	*MAKE A WINNING BOUNCER*	*O*
9th.	*MAKE A WINNING CATCHER*	*O*
10th.	*MAKE A TARGET/GOLFING WINNER*	*O*
11th.	*GOLFING RAMPED UP*	*O*
12th.	*WHEELIE BIN CHIPS OFF THE OLD BLOCK*	*O*
13th.	*WHEELIE BIN ADAPTATIONS*	*O*
14th.	*WATER PISTOL/MARBLE TARGET MIXES*	*O*
15th.	*THE HUMBLE LOO ROLL ENTRANCE*	*O*
16th.	*MARBLE RAMPING IT UP & DOWN*	*O*
17th.	*BE CAREFUL DARTING*	*O*
18th.	*BALLOON/BIN LINERS PARTY TIME*	*B/O*
19th.	*KIDS TARGETED/BAGGED PRIZED MIXES*	*B/O*
20th.	*SPARE BOX IMAGINATION TARGETED WITH INDOOR INTERLUDES*	*I/O*
21st.	*INDOOR COURSE MANAGEMENT (IN CONTROLLED & UNCONTROLLED STAGES!) With a Slalom Interlude) I*	
22nd.	*OUTDOOR LINE PRIZE MANAGEMENT*	*B/O*
23rd.	*OUTDOOR/INDOOR CARD MANIPULATION*	*I/O*
24th.	*JARS: PEANUT BUTTER/HONEY/ PICKLE/JAM*	*I*
25th.	*LETTING OFF STEAM GETTING WET*	*HSG/O*

<u>**PART 2:-**</u>

1st. **YULETIDE > PM EASY DOES IT FOR THE GUEST(S)**   *X*

2nd. **BIRTHDAY:- THAT (POST PARTY) CAKE DETOUR!** *I/O*

3rd. **XMAS > PRIZE DAY PRESENT GUESSING TIME!?**   *I*

4th. **BIRTHDAY > FREE (CHOCOLATE/SWEET) FOR ALL** *O*

5th. **BIRTHDAY > BRING ME A BALL FOR A SWEET GAME** *O*

6th. **+ A JACK & THE GIANT CHALLENGING ESCAPADE!** *O*

7th. **CHRISTMAS > MYA'S CAKE (Part 1 of 2) BAKING**   *X/I*

8th. **CAKE BAKING MYA'S SIMPLE MINGLING MAKING** *X/I*

9th. **SOCIAL GATHERING YOUNG & OLD PRIZE MIXES!** *HSG/O*

10th. **A TEST OF STRENGTH FOR LADIES EYES ONLY (?)** *I/ O*

11th. **CALCULATING & SPELLING CAN BE FUN TOO –
ESPECIALLY AS THERE COULD BE SWEET SUCCESS
GUARANTEED AT THE END!** *I*

12th.   **MIXED PARTY YOUNG & OLD MINGLING TIME – WIN AND
YOU GET FED FIRST!** *I/O*

13th. **MUMMY/DADDY LET'S BAKE A (XMAS) CAKE SURPRISE**   *I*

14th. **CHRISTMAS DAY PRIZE ~~GIVING~~ GUESSING TIME!?**   *I*

15th. **WHY CAR REGISTRATION NUMBERS CAN BE RELAXING** *O/I*

16th. **CHRISTMAS > MYA'S CAKE (Part 2 of 2) COVERING**   *X/ I*

<u>**INTRO:**</u>

**If there is one thing,
having to stay cooped up,
<u>*for so long*</u>, at home together
has taught us –
How inventive we must become
to keep those around us occupied!
And it is not only the kids,
but the adult kids at heart too!
And those who need to be
educated in how
'<u>*to have simple fun!*</u>'**

**<u>But, this is primarily directed
At the parents!</u>
Who might also
'Make the(ir)own Recycling Difference
<u>Although,
You might not want the kids getting
Too many ideas at adapting this
Too much to their boisterous
Uncontrolled way!</u>
NB All photo/picture contributors are fully
acknowledged...
But, for now, it's special thanks <u>to</u>
<u>ALL OF YOU!!!</u>**

So, **<u>Dad & Mum</u>**, let's start with this 'sporty' caption:-

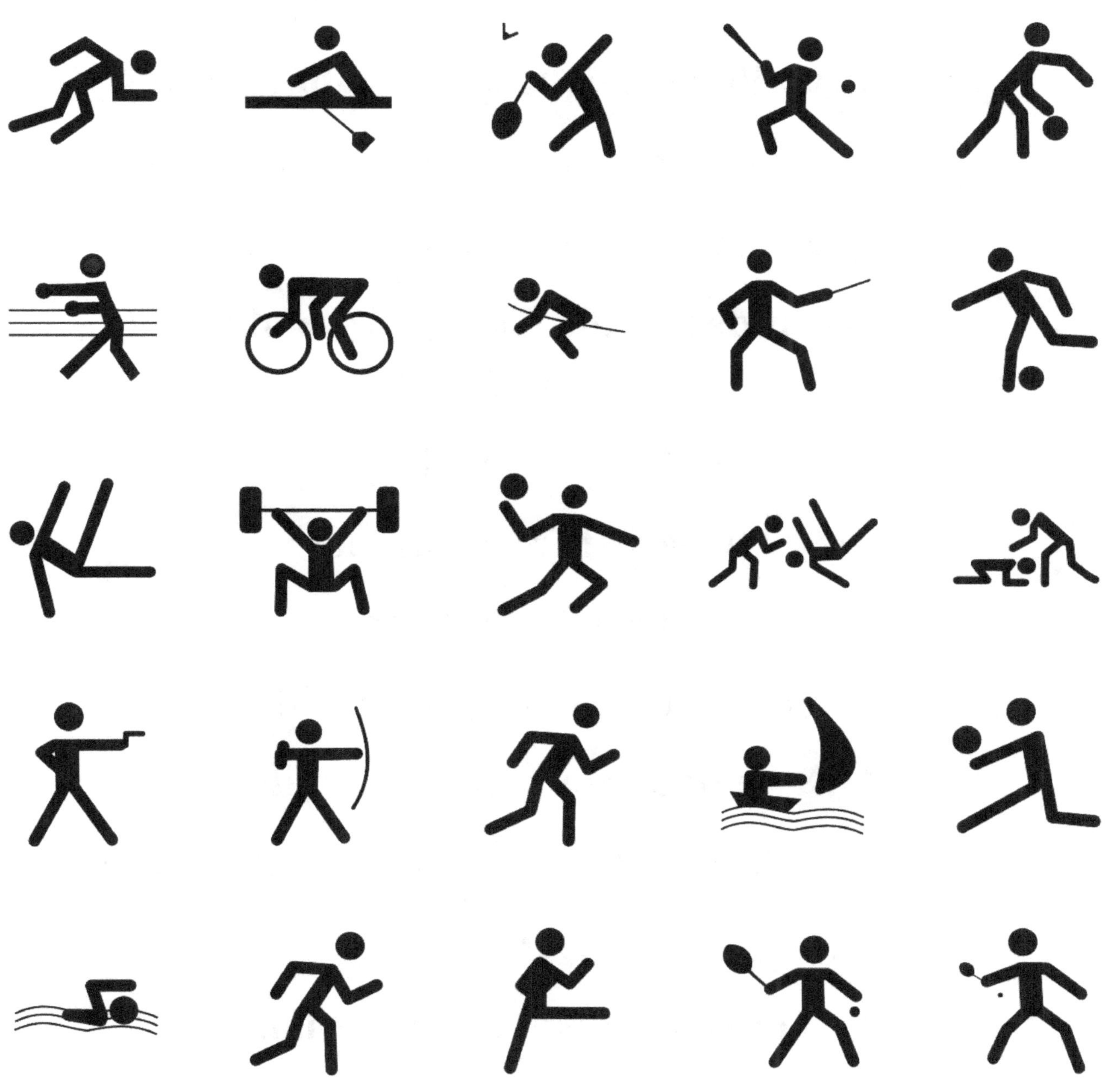

<u>I have tried my best throughout the book to highlight what might be dangerous for kids; the rest is up to you! So, you adults/carers out there, remember it's you, not I, who has to bear the responsibility for any accidents on your watch!</u>

Yes it does look like:-

Something out of the Olympics?

But, ours will have to be our own backyard style

– with what we can find to amuse us all!

And, yes, I said all, as all the family can play:-

Old Grandad to the young 6 year old twins,
Johnny/Jenny.

In these strained times,

the great fresh outdoors

has a lot to offer,

as do reject/remnant household items

in addition to those found

lying gathering dust in the garage &/or loft:

<u>ALL</u>

offer great source material!

<u>**So, first:-**</u>

It's Back to Selection Basics:
- **What have we at our immediate disposal?**
- **So many can be adapted for play**
- **And here they are >>>**
- **And they should be around, even if just hand-me-downs!**
- **And they won't break your personal savings bank!**

<u>**But they're not used in the conventional way!?**</u>

Your availability list, at your disposal, could go something like this:-

<u>**HOUSEHOLD PLAYTHINGS:-**</u>

<u>**So, in no particular order –**</u>
<u>**What can we expect to find about us?**</u>

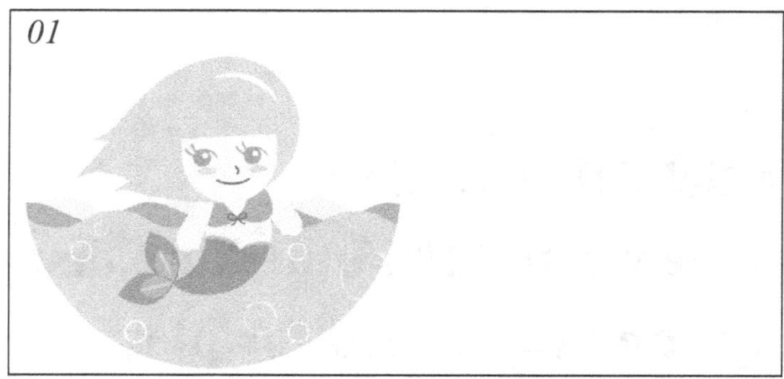

*Yes, admittedly, we all don't possess one, or if we did and not use it, as likely it would have a hole in it and not retain the water – if this is the case, fix it, or if not we have an alternative '**box**' below.*

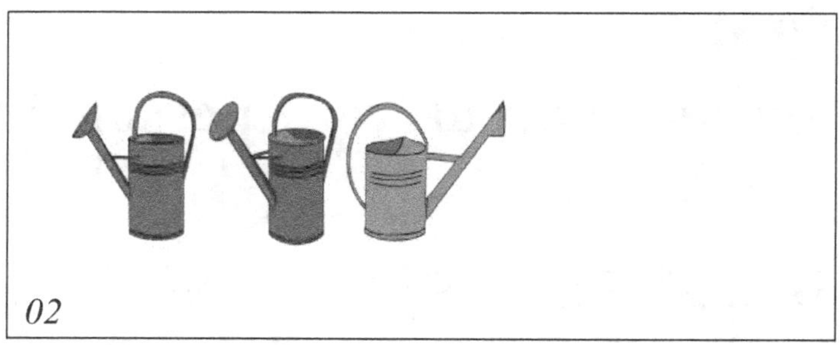

They come in different sizes and as likely yours will have its rose/sprinkler missing – no worry, as it is the area where the water goes in & not out which we'll need!

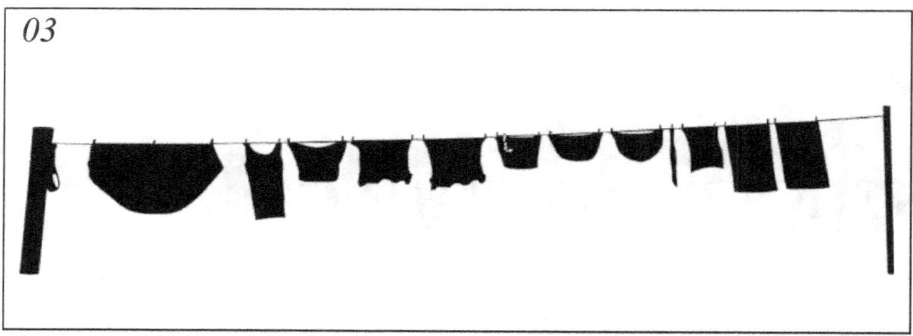

The washing line (the longer the better in some instances below), but the pegs not so much.

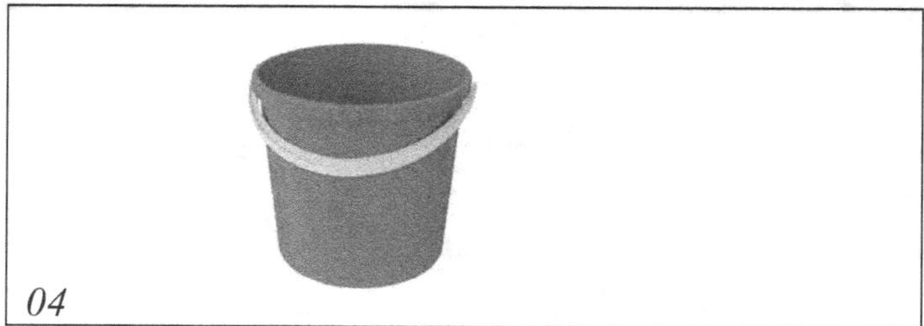

Buckets come in so many shapes & sizes: if yours has a broken handle, no matter, as we don't need carry anything in it and use it standing on the floor as above, or inverted too!

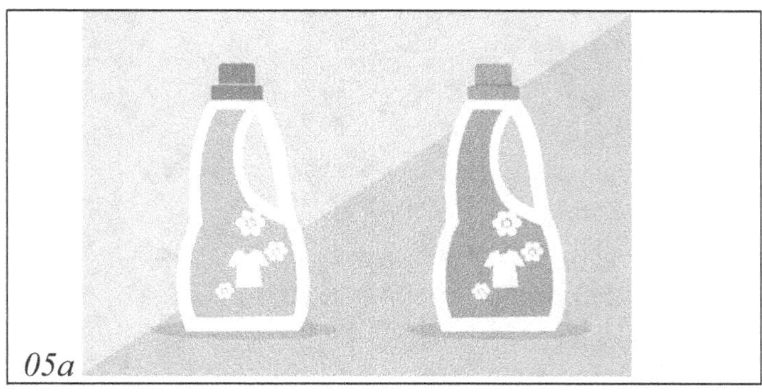

Plastic washing up bottles + *Shampoo & Shower* + **Fairy Pod Child Proof Containers even the humble used toilet roll (Later)...**
We throw away after use, regrettably, as they are a great source of fun in various ways.

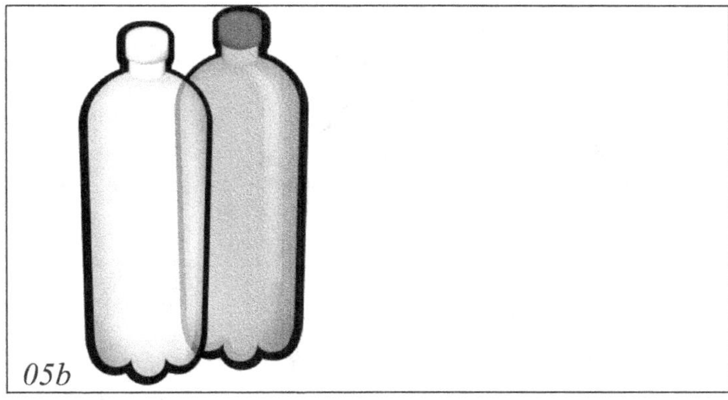

Like above, we throw these after use, regrettably, as they are a great source of fun in various ways.

No, I don't expect you to have one lying about in the back garden/garage/shed, but the picture significance is how we can simply create ramp systems for games.

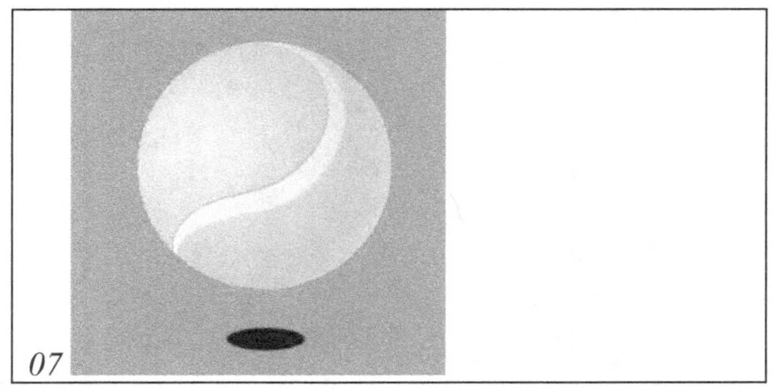

I'm sure, well hope, you have a supply of these around – the quality is immaterial.

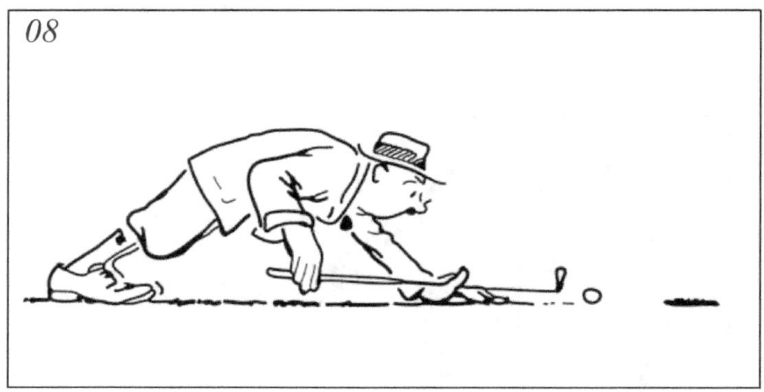

Again the caption is misleading, but if you remember what I have in store is for all ages, even Grandpa can play golf, although what follows later, will mean hell be playing far more than that! But, for our fun time all we need is the putter and possibly a wedge (or lofted iron please).

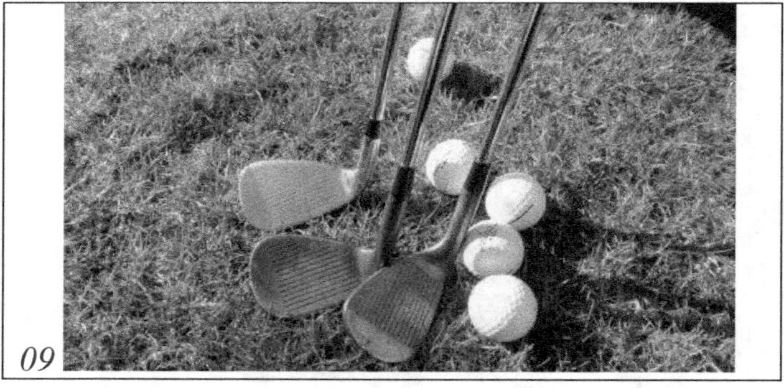

Continuing the ball theme, here the humble golf ball which as a youngster I and some friends would always try to recover those in water hazards and sell them back to Club Members, getting soaking wet was par for our ball retrieving course! Ha! Excuse the pun!

BUT CARE THEY ARE VERY HARD! AND GLASS/WINDOWS ARE

NO MATCH-PLAY FOR THEM!

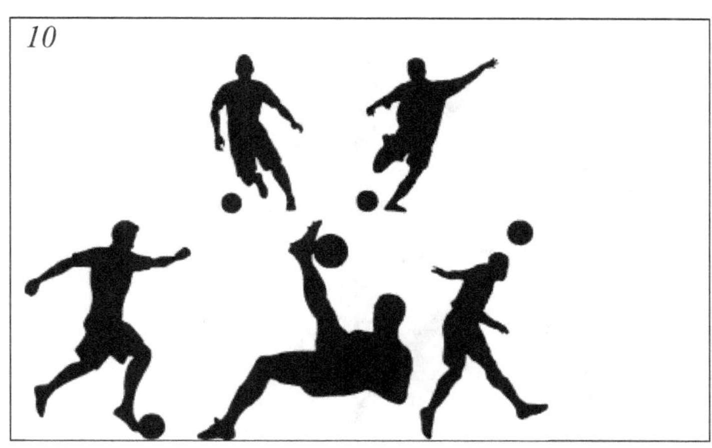

All youngsters now seem to play soccer/football and some are very adept at the game possessing great skill for their age; even at a tender 8 they (Boy & Girl) can run rings around their mother and grand-parents, but not good old Dad, unless he lets them! But the Wheelie Bin might later have a great say in the matter.

BUT HAVE SOME CARE AS SOME BALLS ARE HARDER THAN OTHERS!

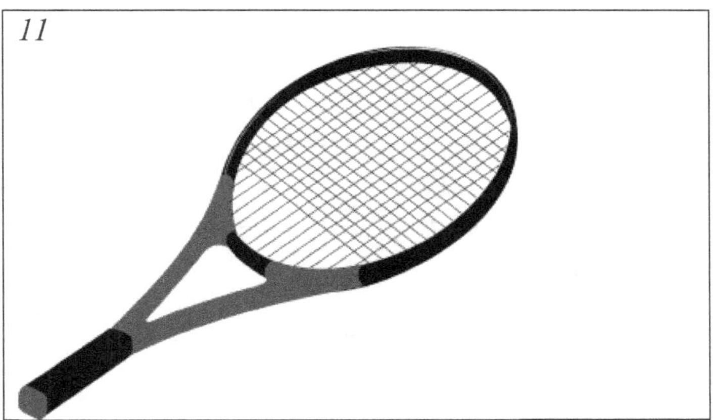

Unless you have a budding Federer in the family, again I imagine we all have some old racquet or two in the deep recesses of our attic/garage, or shed: the quality is not important and it adds to the fun!

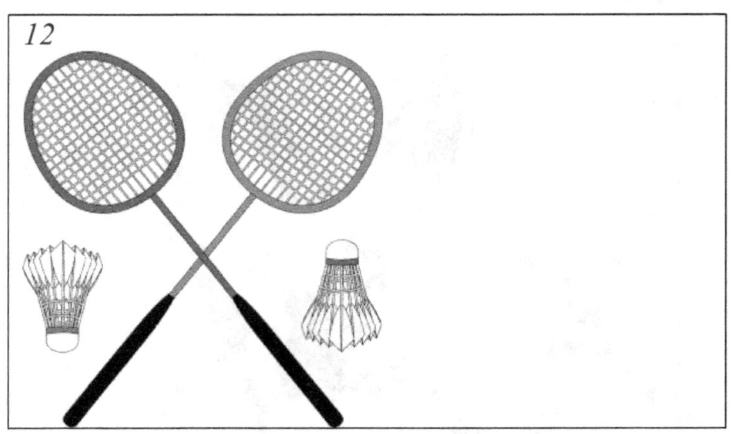

Here the old garden stand-by, but for me the drawback is the strength of the wind which can spoil the game – below, it is an enjoyable extra skill element factor, or just a plain family laughing matter!

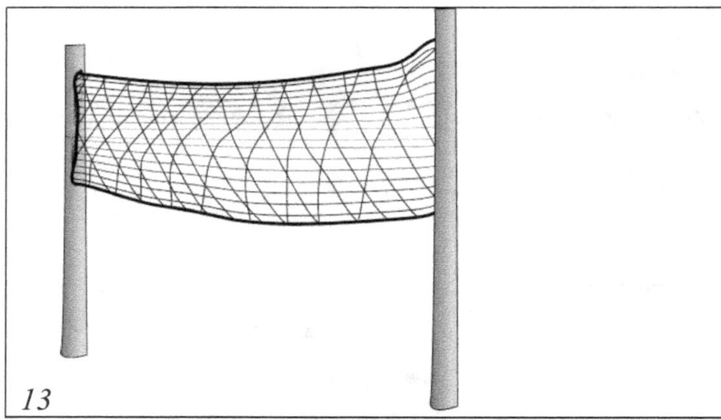

The net at the right level is something which not all have, but here it is not material as games can be adapted around its height, or lack of it.

There are 3 captions devoted to this sport as the more shuttles the better. And once again, quality is something we are not fussed about!

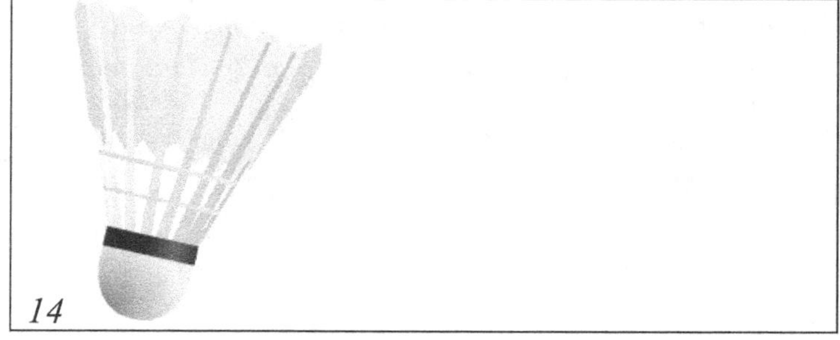

Can be played in the Sun, or Rain depending how adventurous you feel?

The usual problem with the next sport, like badminton above, is the wind factor, apart from setting the fiddly net up!

But, Above & Below, the net is not required, just one bat at times +t a few balls are far better than one!

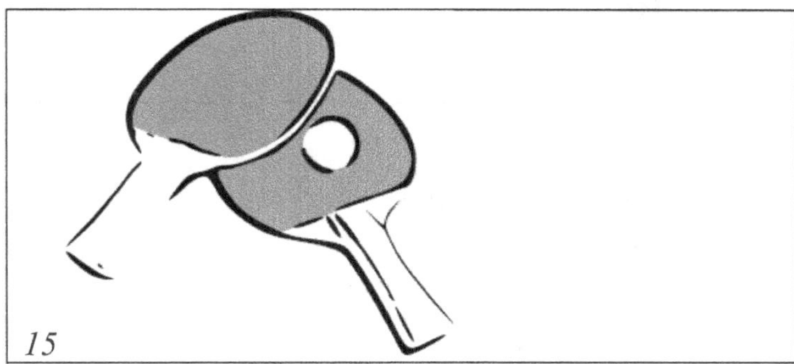

Yes, not ideal when windy, but perhaps if the object is not just making it bounce on the other side?

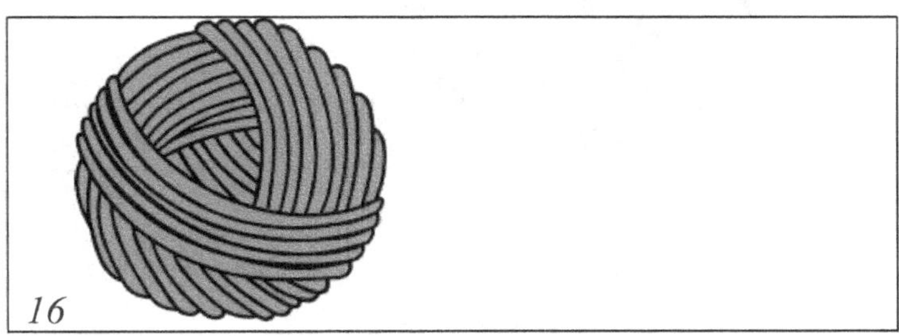

You'll find string has a number of fun uses (No not tying up Dad!) – Although the caption could just have been a ball of wool (But make sure you get Nan's permission!

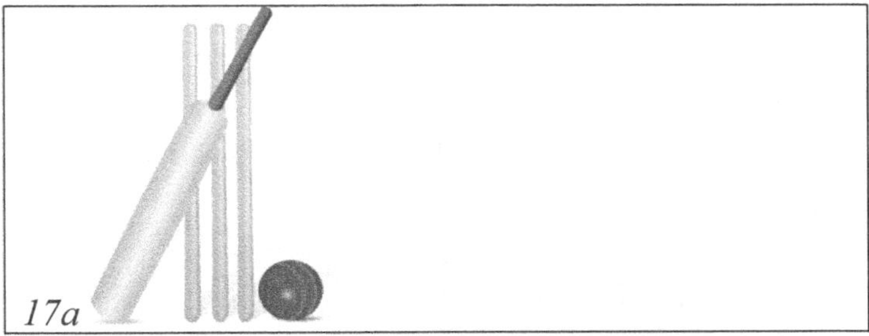

This caption is for the stumps, which can be supplemented by Granny's knitting needles (below), or Dad's screwdrivers. And here is the first of my many cautionary notes: these can be dangerous to people's health, in silly-prankish hands: so use them strictly supervised. If in doubt leave them out!

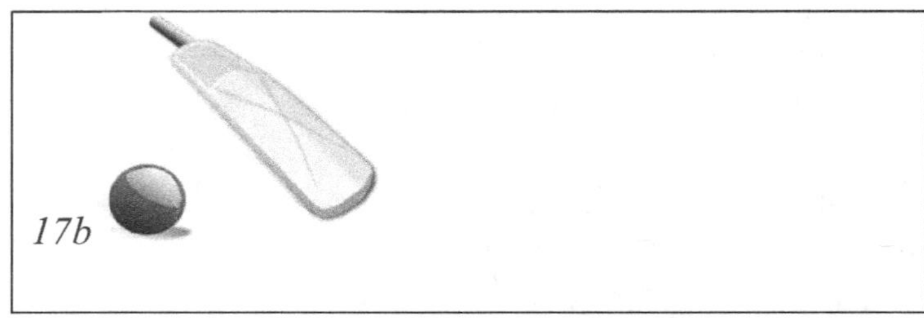

So, we have the bat & ball, the latter another most dangerous item to health and next door's property: so cricket balls are taboo! The bat will be handy for other softer substitutes.

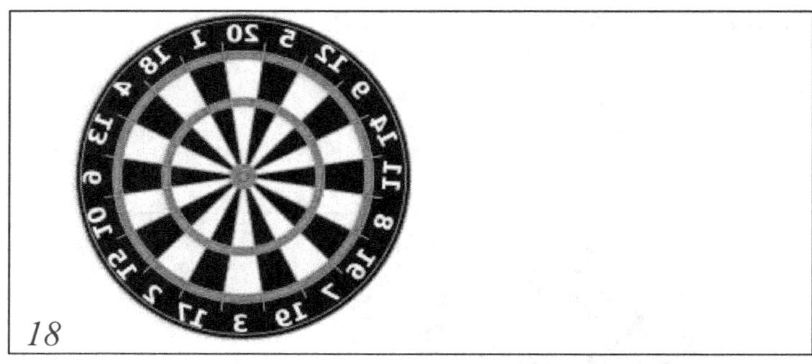

A simple dart board, without the darts, for obvious reasons: they can kill. For me fortunately in my errant youth they didn't! (Below – you have been warned!)

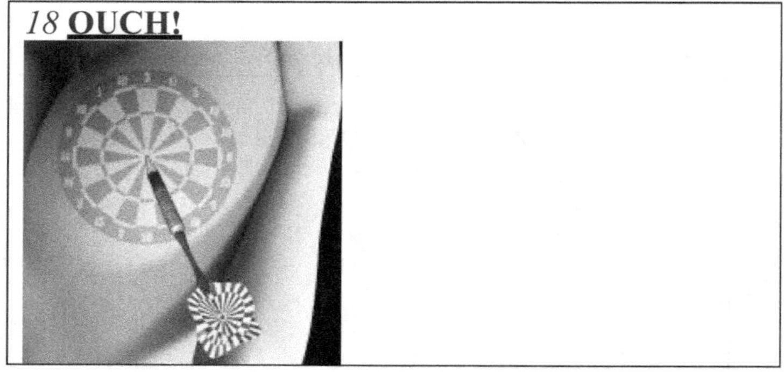

Following on from above, this 'created' picture might raise a few sniggers, but the message is plain and clear I hope to all parents, if you use the darts like the game(s) below, no playing about – serious stuff then! Otherwise there would be bloody consequences as there were with my 'wrist' incident! But those were 'apparently' the good old unsupervised post war 50s & 60s!

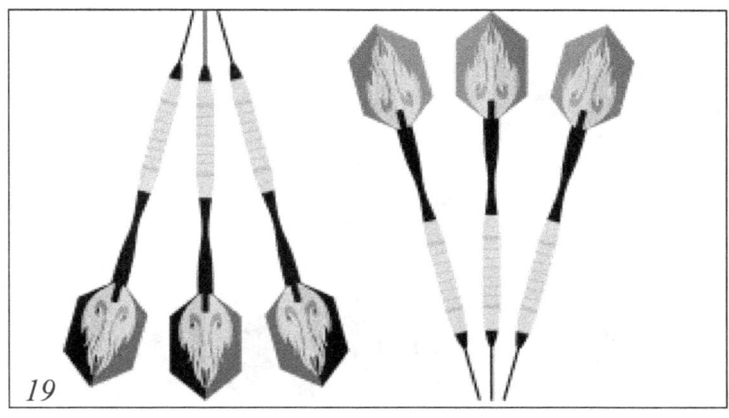

So, above, are the items we handle with ~~kid~~ adult supervised gloves!

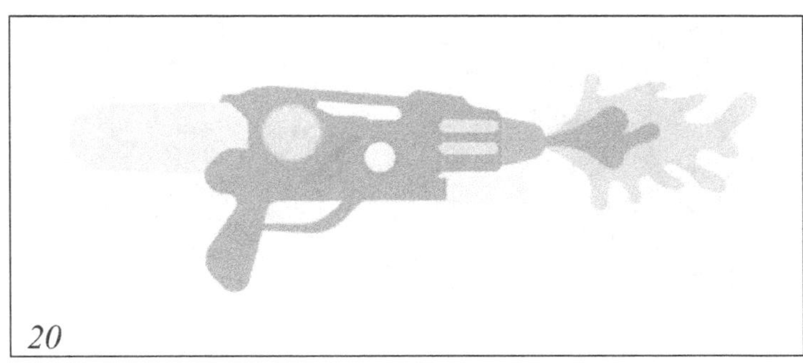

Now, back to something innocuous, although not if you're sprayed as you garden-sunbathe!
But, indiscriminate firing will not be the order of the day!

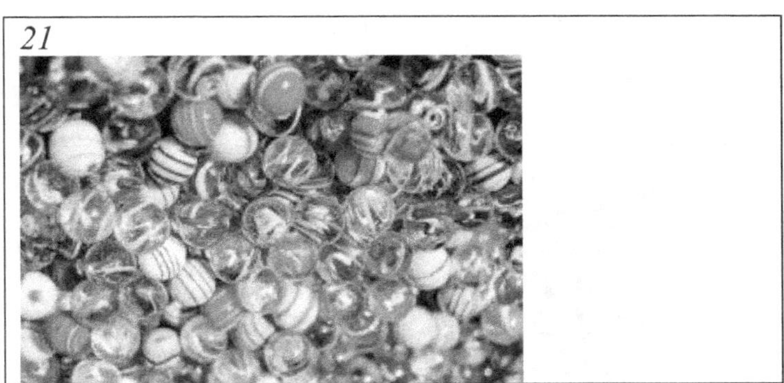

Again in the old 50s/60s these were a street game past-time, but can easily be adapted to a garden
skill game for all!

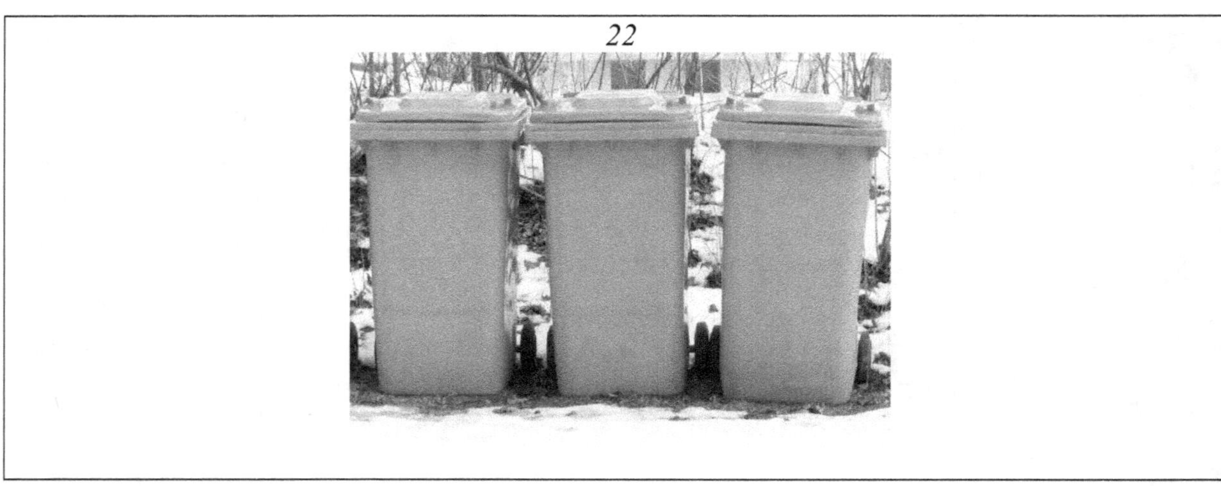

Here, this Winter Christmas Caption to show potentially the more the merrier! Ho! Ho! Ho!

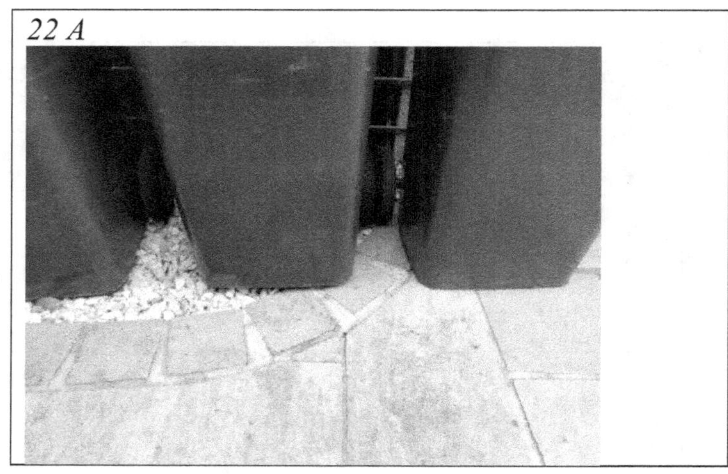

22 A

The picture is to show how the humble wheelie bin can be adapted for fun gaming: here if you look closely just the right size for trying to putt those golf balls?

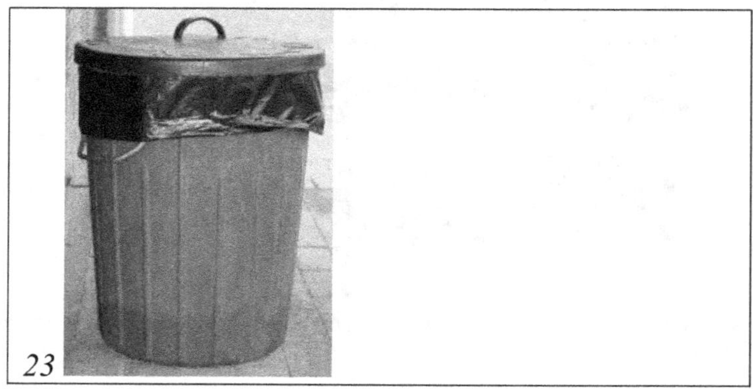

23

Here the message is starkly simple: those bins can be the source of dirt/germs etc so best to line them first before your kids start scrambling in/around them!

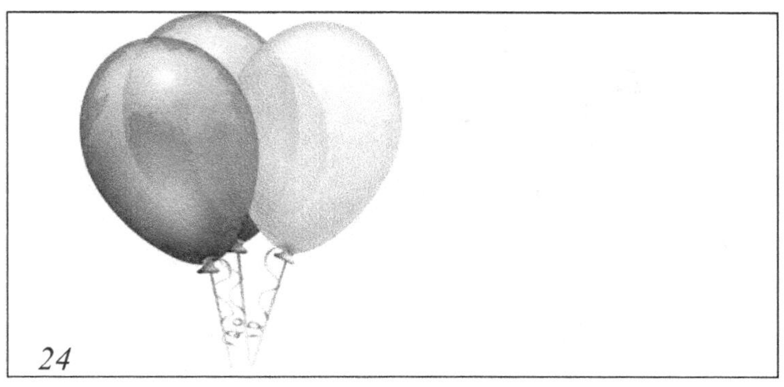

Balloons for outside games? Surely they'll fly all over the place? Not if you??????

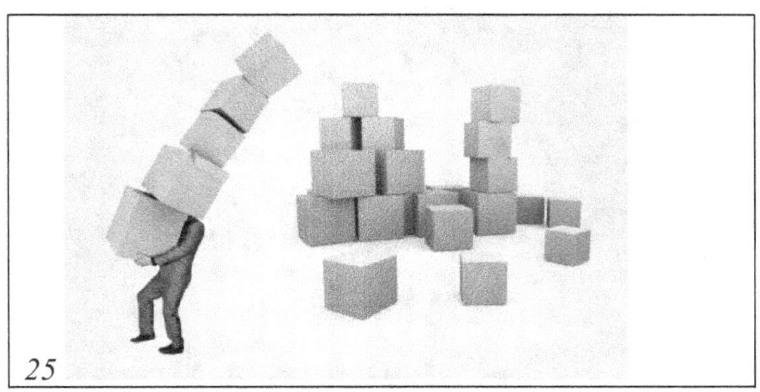

(Amazon?) Delivery anybody? Well make sure you keep all the boxes, no matter the sizes! You never can imagine how much fun youngsters can be given by Daddy's simple use of scissors & tape!

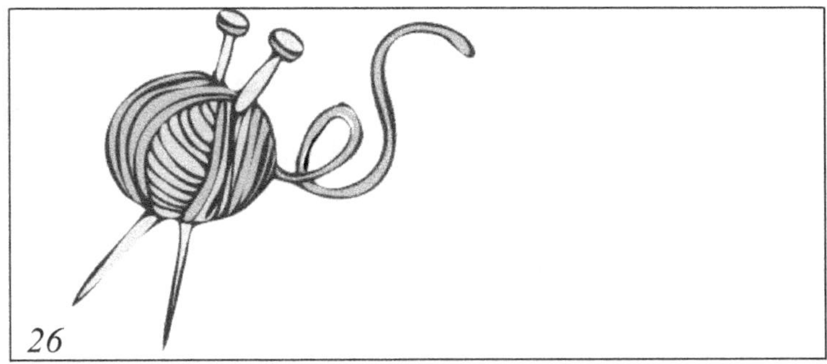

Just to re-iterate <u>warnings</u> use them as substitutes but knitting needles point down and out of sight at all times! Unlike the caption above.

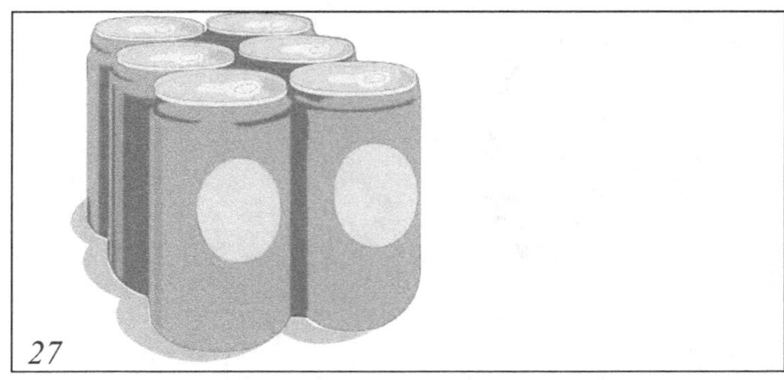

Similar to the plastic bottles at the top, but with the added bonus of being so lightweight.

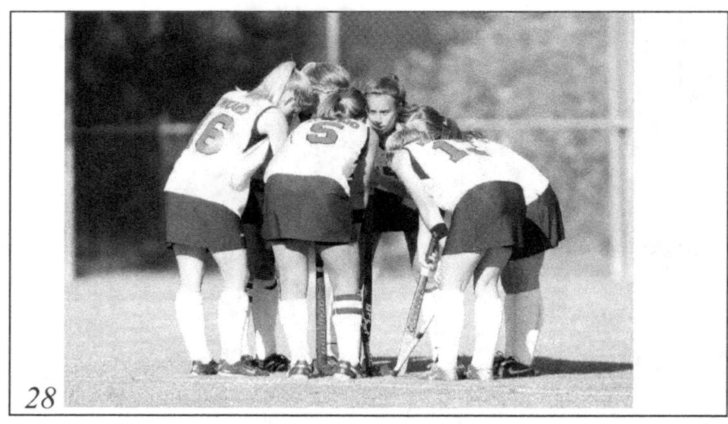

Couldn't resist this picture as a reminder to me as I forgot about this sport initially, that you out there might have a boy/girl who play this game – so hockey sticks might also be lying about in your garage/shed too? They'll also be a match for the English Cricket Bat, or Golf Putter later!

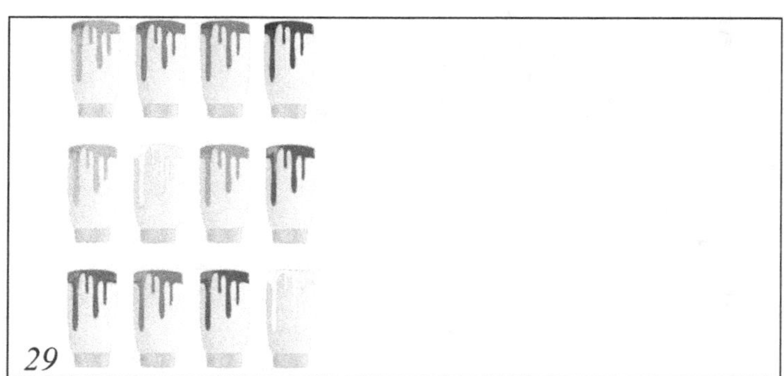

Surely you'll all have a supply of these half empty on garage /shed floors – they are ideal as perfect solid obstacles!

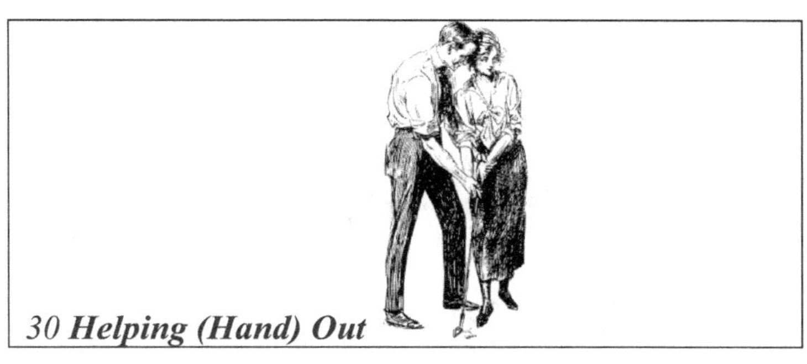

30 Helping (Hand) Out

Like the old grandad golf picture before it, there is a message for all, that the fun is for all and all might not be totally adept at what they are expected to do and so will need a helping hand. Failing this make sure the sides have a certain balance to them, otherwise introduce your own unique handicap system1

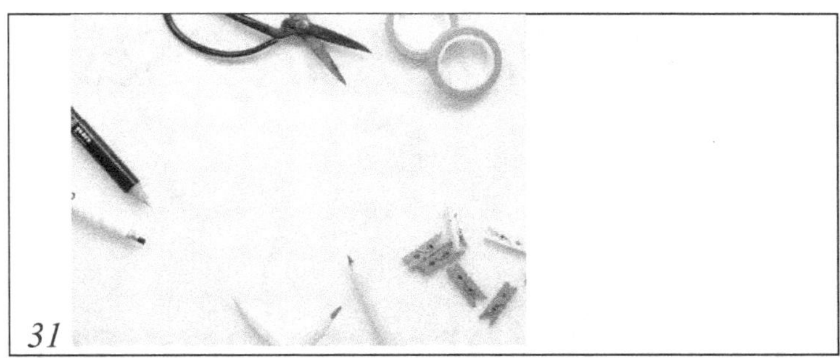

31

I put Jess's photo here as a reminder that there are other items about the house, like at work stations, where those old stand-byes like scissors/tape/clips etc can be found which might assist the games set up.

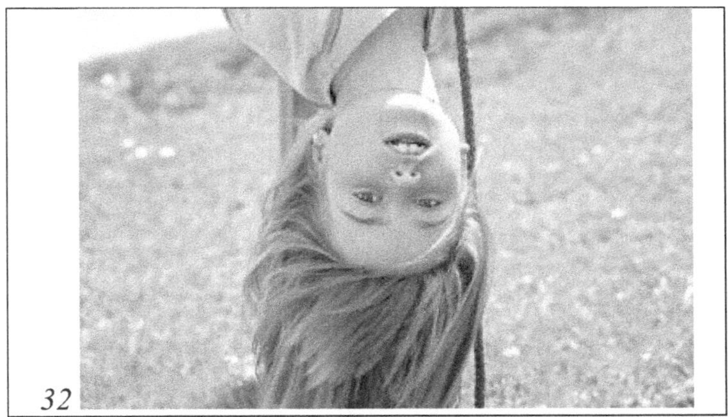

32

And lastly, for the moment, with pride of place here is an >

Upside-Down *who'll be introduced much later into MY Card Game*

<u>YOUR PLAYLIST ↓</u>

<u>SO FROM ABOVE WE HAVE:- ></u>

1. *Kiddies Paddling Pool*

2. *Watering Cans*

3. *Washing Lines*

4. *Buckets*

5. *A) Used Washing Up Plastic Bottles*

5. *B) Used Plastic Drinks Bottles*

6. *Ramp (incl. cardboard/hardboard)*

7. *Tennis balls, or any similarly sized type, even plastic with holes in!*

8. *Golf Clubs = Putter + Iron/wedge (Not the Driver!)*

9. *Golf balls (But care how hard they're hit!)*

10. *Footballs Hard &Soft*

11. *Tennis rackets*

12. *Badminton rackets*

13. *Badminton Net*

14. *Shuttlecocks*

15. *Table Tennis Bats + Ping Pong Balls*

16. *Ball of string*

17. *Cricket bat + stumps (No cricket balls!)*

18. *Dart board*

19. *Darts (With a use Warning from above)*

20. *Water pistols*

21. *Marbles (Remember these are hard, too!)*

22. *Wheelie Bins*

23. *Wheelie Bin Liners*

24. *Balloons (Fun might be the blowing up?)*

25. *Delivery/Packing Boxes*

26. *Knitting Needles Point Down↓ (Without Any Doubt!)+ball of wool*

27. *Cans (used)*

28. *Hockey Stick*

29. *Paint Pots (Tightly Shut!*

30. *Family Handicap Assistance*

31. *Scissors/Tape/Etc...*

32. *Upside Down Card Fun*

32. a *Card(s) Choices Generally Adapted*

33. *Lacrosse*

34. *Honey jar/pot*

35. *Peanut Butter Jar*

The Choice of Sweets is Entirely Yours!

And, so, as wonderfully as

I can make it,

Here are the games

I play with those

Who really are made for them!

I hope you know

Many who do, too!

<u>ENJOY</u>

Regards, Michael YR Xavier.

<u>BUT, FIRST COME THE DISSENTERS >>>></u>

But, and it is just a small But, that your garden area is too small?

But, and it is just a small But, that you only have a lawn garden?

But, and it is just a small But, that you only have a paved garden?

But, and it is just a small But, that your garden is not flat?

But, and it is just a small But, that your lawn is broken up by shrubs?

But, and it is just a small But, that your garden is on different levels?

But, and it is just a small But, that you don't want the garden dug up?

"A mere Bagatelle," = *A thing regarded as too unimportant or easy to be worth much consideration* **as my Father used to say.**

You never know till you've tried!

HERE THE FUN FINALLY BEGINS:

But, *Dear Parents/Carers* now to the real game reasons for writing this Book – Perhaps A.K.A. Fun on a Discovered Shoe String?

So, have you ever considered?

Intro to 'A' Game(s):-

A.   Inter-Family/Friends/Relatives Games of Skill?

But, and it is just a BIG But, ensure there is always a prize, no matter how small, at the end of each game. AND, skilful little Johnny must not be allowed to win everything, so it pays to change his sides for different events.

NB Age is not significant here, so long as the teams are well balanced – competitively!

Here you will (from experience?) need to determine the best distance between contestants and target, as there will be varying ages and skill levels taking part.
It helps enormously that 'Daddy' is handicapped the most – <u>poor Dad</u>,
&/or he is mostly partnered by Mum versus the Kids – though you know your family best, so make up your own teams, or plain individuals.
For throwing/accuracy games suggest 10 # attempts is the norm!

Similarly, if a game of skill, like golf, make 10 # the maximum a person can be scored!

KNOCK 'EM OVER:

(Here Two Indoor & Out)

- Fairy-Thee-Well 6/10 Pin Bowling ###
  - Thinking of 5 & 6 above collect your old & used Washing Up Liquid Bottles and create your own Tennis Ball Bowling Alley in your Back Yard &/or Home Hallway!
  - You can play the conventional 2 shot game or how many it takes to knock them all over, with a maximum they can take #.
  - You can also stipulate that those knocked over are taken away from the pack.
  - There again, you could just leave them where they fell!
  - You can make the game easier, or more difficult by the distance between pins
- Fairy-Thee-Well _'Timber'_ Tower Tumbling
  - The _timber_ reference is to the warning call lumberjacks shout out as a tree is about to fall...you can introduce this for the kids to shout out as they accomplish their game's task
  - Here Fairy Washing Machine Pod Containers fit the game(s) bill admirably
  - You can make the towers either one tall single one and see how many goes it takes to make it tumble over.

- Or you can have them 2 high & upwards and let your tennis ball destroy what it can
- But here I would just add a scoring note: at times the container is not knocked over, although it is knocked out of its original placement – so to avoid arguments use chalk to mark underneath the X spot from which it must be moved from!
- Although you could allow a bonus point if totally knocked over – up to you
- You can adapt and create 1 &/or 2 pyramid(s) from 3 &/or 6 – the knocking out/down/overrule(s) above could also apply
- All above with a maximum #they can take
- Perhaps consider some sweet tempting to get them playing – one on each container – knock it off to win it!

NB ### *If you venture down to your local supermarket with the kids I am sure, if you set them this task, they'll relish the challenge: they'll discover, as they go round, that there are many alternatives, which could be used as a ten pin substitute –*

Here are just those I noticed wandering around > Pringle containers and the Supermarket own versions; Hellman's Mayonnaise/HP Sauce/Heinz Ketchup/the inner cardboard tube of your kitchen paper/Quality Street/Cadbury's Celebrations/Roses Chocolates/There is even something purpose built, if you consider Califia Farm's own Oat Creamer range....

The list is Ever-Expansive Not Expensive! Unless you <u>Count</u> the <u>Countless</u> Wine/Whisky Bottle Tube Holders!

Now onwards to the other A1 ideas!!!

MAKE A WINNING SPLASH:

A1a And so, from the list above, let's start with something not all you have – that elusive paddling pool – and let's use the following:

1, Paddling Pool 7, Balls 8, Golf Clubs 9, Golf balls 10, Footballs

11, Tennis rackets 12, Badminton rackets

13, Badminton Net 14, Shuttlecocks

15, Table Tennis Bats + Ping Pong Balls

17. Cricket bat + stumps (+ 21 Marbles see end alternative?)

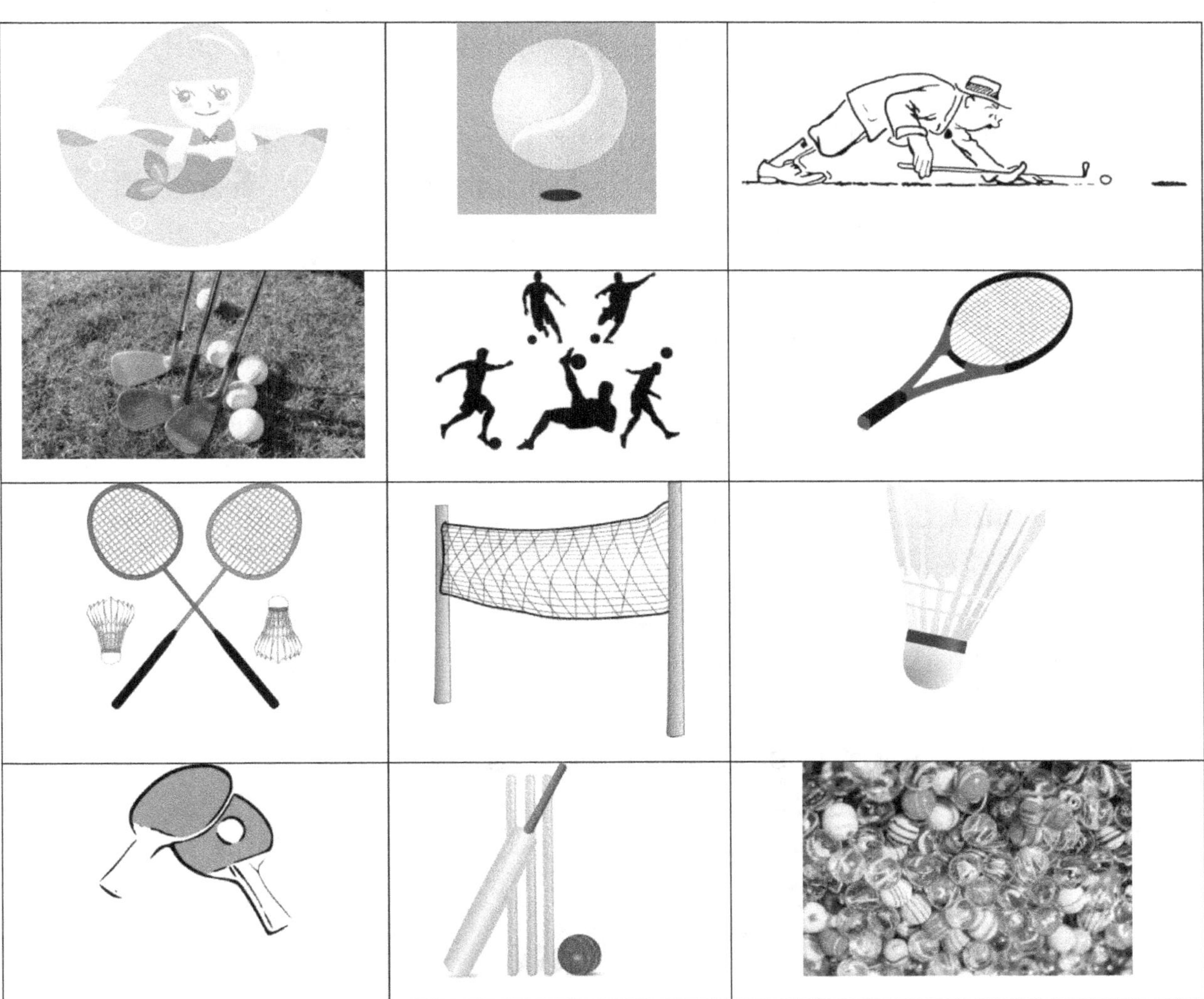

So, we fill the pool up with water – say half full – then it is a case of how many we get inside!

- With the tennis racquet the individual can do it themselves, or get their partner to toss them the tennis ball to hit;

- The same can be done with the cricket bat and tennis ball (A cricket ball WILL be a might too brave of you & too costly for you, in view of the danger of damage to property/selves/others!) So, simply put **Cricket Balls are taboo** unless used in place of tennis/golf balls as part of an obstacle/golf course (A5i below).

- With the golf club the individual can try to chip his golf ball into the pool. However, if you only have a putter, then create a ramp to drive upward and onward! The pool has water to stop balls jumping out, this is particular applicable to the golf ball!

- Use of the badminton equipment is restricted by any windy weather, but, when calm, string the net across above head height between striker & pool and try to loop the shuttle into the water.

- You substitute the ping pong bats for racquets as another game.

- The teams make up/number of attempts/points system/prize system are all up to you – but limit the size and number of the last named: we don't want to run out of our bribe element.

- As a smaller alternative marbles can be tossed instead - When the coast is clear – that goes without saying!

- Nothing to hit the balls with? Ask Mum who knows where the pots and pans are!

OFF YOU GO TRY ME

MAKE A FOOTBALL SPLASH:

A1b And, so, for the football fanatics, who want to make a big splash, here is your opportunity:

We only need *1, Paddling pool 7, balls + 10, (heavy) Football* with the pool full to the brim.

Balls mean sweet prizes, so simply ask the competitors in turns, the youngest first, to kick/chip the footballs into the pool to win a prize (Or best accumulative score wins say 2 sweets to any/all losers one sweet each!)

To add fun to the game, depending who is willing: Dad yes, Mum certainly not, as it means going behind the Paddling Pool, getting splashed &/or wet stopping the Football flying past (Into the neighbour's garden?)

OFF YOU GO TRY ME

MAKE A WINNING BOUNCER:

A2i So, we have dispensed with the pool, but only for an interlude while, so don't empty it!

The next game type, more sedate, but certainly more difficult – if difficulty is what you want - is using the following:

2, Watering Cans 4, Buckets 15 Table Tennis (balls & bats).

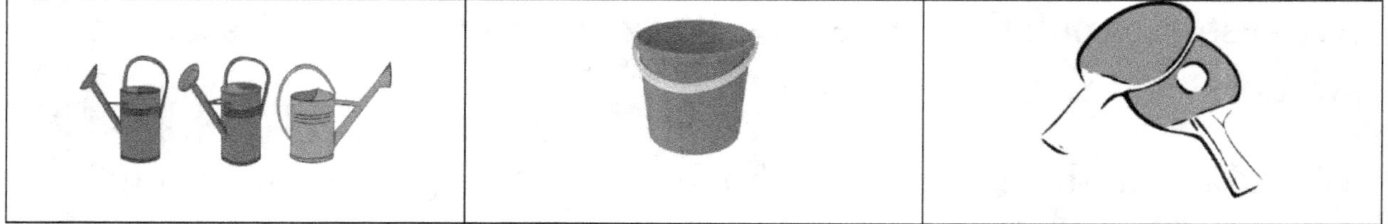

Here is a perfect example where the handicapping the best player – good ole Dad – has the more difficult assignment.

He has to hit the ping pong ball into the watering can, via its half-sized opening; the lesser lights & Mum have the bucket as their full-sized opening target!

The distance determined might be more miss than hit!

ALTHOUGH:- From a few pages back > for concrete paved areas:

? Ask Mum who knows where the pots and pans are!

Using the bounce test, get a few pots/saucepans and lay them out. Then challenge the players to see how many balls they can bounce into the pots/pans.

Here it *fun-helps* to then have the pots/pans on varying levels!

It also helps avoid the possibly regularly bounce out scenario!

OFF YOU GO TRY ME

A2ii A combination of **1 & 2** using the Buckets & Tennis Balls.

Here we set the bucket to our side and try to throw the ball against a wall in front of us and try to make it bounce into the bucket!

Too difficult?

So, as a supposed easier option, place the bucket(s) away from you, sufficiently to allow a bounce between you and them.

Then toss them into the bucket making sure the ball bounces at least once before hitting its mark! The game can be extended by incrementally increasing the distance in between, by say a foot/100cm at a time, up to 10 feet (+ 3 metres).

Here, paving stones are more likely to maintain the bounce accuracy, rather than some uneven grassed areas?

OFF YOU GO TRY ME

ALTHOUGH:- From a few pages back > for concrete paved areas:

? Ask Mum who knows where the pots and pans are!

Using the bounce test, get a few pots/saucepans and lay them out.
Then challenge the players to see how many balls they can bounce into the pots/pans.
Here it _fun-helps_ to then have the pots/pans on varying levels!
It also helps avoid the possibly regularly bounce out scenario!

OFF YOU GO TRY ME

MAKE A WINNING CATCHER:

A3 A simple play practised incessantly by the professionals:

Dad hits the tennis ball in the air, say 10 times, and each other individual, _in turn_, tries to catch it the most – usually 2 handed.

If you have a small family unit of parents + two kids (a boy & a girl) then you can play the older child + the mother x the team made up of the younger + father.

You can ramp it up a notch demanding the catchers use just their good hand.

Then, yes you've guessed it, insist they only use their bad hand!

Continuing the catching theme – likely there will have been excuses as Daddy didn't toss it well enough etc... Then, here with the next there can be only the self-thrower to blame!

With their usual 10 attempts make each person thrown the ball in the air, pirouette a full 180 degrees and catch the ball on the descent.

Vary this by insisting the ball bounces At Least once!

Needless to say play on grass, definitely not concrete paving!

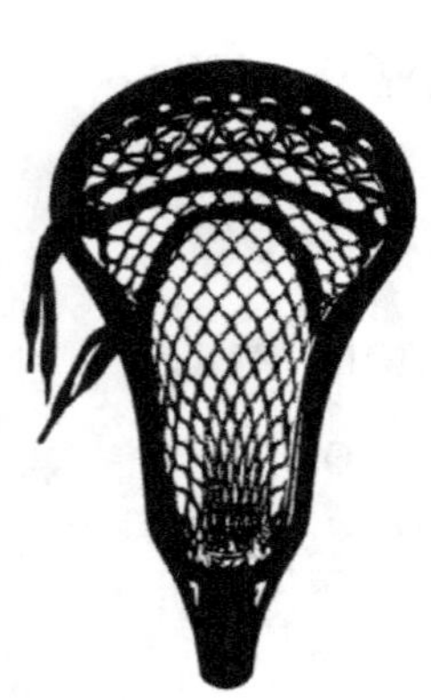

And for the American **Lacrosse** Players, _something out of Alien:- >33_ This could have been introduced earlier above, but it will do just as well here: lend your stick (head) out and rather than the normal game catching style, toss the ball up and people catch it at horizontal, rather than the 45 degree/virtual vertical 90 degree level. Continue with the toss in the air pirouette etc...

Leave the fast hand speed passing/shooting for the playing field, or perhaps not? (See e.g. A4 Below).

OFF YOU GO TRY ME

MAKE A TARGET/GOLFING WINNER:

A4 Continuing the required accuracy theme, we need:

5a & b, Used Washing Up/ Drinks Bottles/Cans 7, Balls

8, Golf Clubs 9, Golf balls 11, Tennis rackets

17 Cricket Bat 27 Cans (used)

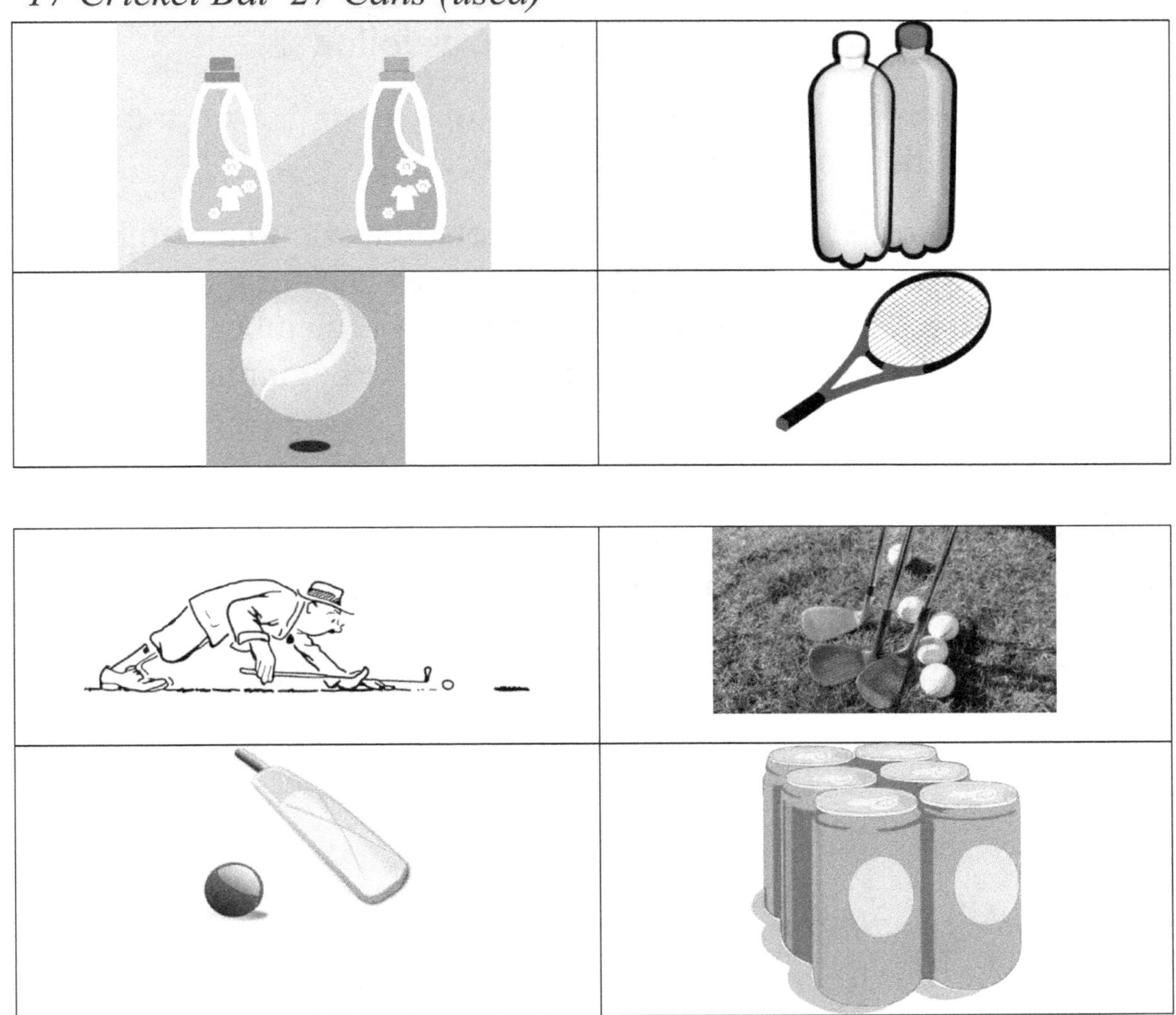

Way 1: Set up your targets *5a & b, 27,* plastic bottles/cans/cartons some way from you in haphazard fashion.

Then using *7, 8, 9, 11, 17,* each <u>in a designated order</u>, see how many can be hit. These should ensure many rounds.

NB Best if you only use the putter, <u>not the wedge</u> - yes?

I have purposely excluded the footballs – we don't want it to be too easy and done with!

A point for each object struck, after which it is taken out of the equation.

<u>**Way 2:**</u> If you want it to be a game, being fought to the finish, arrange the scoring in a somewhat novel fashion, as follows:-

 If you have say 6 targets, score the first one hit as 1, working upwards to 6 for the last one knocked over!

Smarties/Liquorice-Allsorts/Haribo sweets, for example, can be the equivalent winning prize. But, if the youngest is having no joy, let him/her move a foot closer after each round – remember then to ensure the objects are at least 9 feet away at the beginning, at least!

OFF YOU GO TRY ME

A5 And here, now a less aggressive, perhaps more skilful version? Or, so the grandparents would have the kids believe/!

So, you set up your targets *5a & b,* plastic bottles/cartons some way from you in golf course fashion and using only *8, 9,* or failing this *7, 17.*

(Here I must apologise to the female Hockey Players of this world there might be a Hockey Stick, 28 hanging about to use instead of the Cricket Bat (Not all the World Play the Game!
Nor Cricket, you'd reply!
Yes, sorry! I'm British!)

Then, in pairs, or individually, see how many strokes it takes you to complete the course.

OFF YOU GO TRY ME

<u>But there is one important Golf Thing Missing?</u>

A5i) But, hey, there are no holes; yes, so it's just a case of knocking [X] against, or over, the bottle/can to complete the hole and re-erect for your opponent, as you continue to the next! [X] Here Dad is the Judge!

Your tee of is adjacent the last bottle/can you struck/knocked over.

The glory of this is that you can get items from the garage/store shed to use as *obstacles*, to make the course more demanding#!

29 the *Paint Pots (Tightly Shut!)*, a typical example here, or *25* the *Delivery/Packing cardboard boxes*!

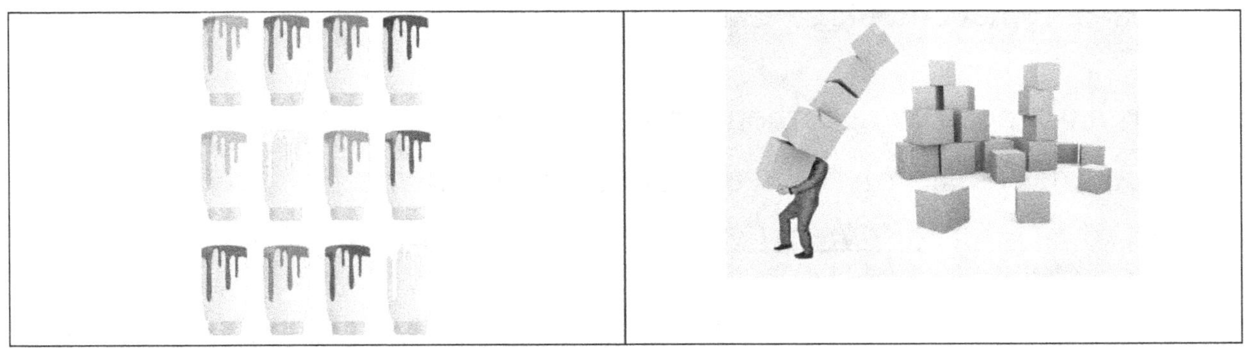

And change the course layout continually thereafter! It's amazing how long your 18 Tee Golf Course will take to complete, before the sweet prizes are handed out.

Again remember the littlest one should have say a stroke per hole advantage. But, even with this he/she cannot win/share a hole make sure there is a prize for last place!

OFF YOU GO TRY ME

GOLFING RAMPED UP:

A5ii) ***If, you are able to dig out a hole, the more the better***.

Here, then you introduce more realism, then, the golf balls come into their own.

Forewarning: But also <u>make sure your hole is big enough to accommodate the hand</u> taking the ball out of the hole!

Those not wishing to dig more than one hole, the simple solution, with using just the one, is the changing of the tee-off area with the ever changing placement of various obstacle items!

You might even consider using the water filled pool, or any other type obstacle like the paint pots/buckets/ boxes etc to chip over – so you'll need both types of club wedge/lofted iron PLUS putter, or hockey stick as a replacement, eh girls?

If you have no *9* wedge, then we need adapt plank of wood, or hardboard, OR simply folded/supported cardboard *25* placed on a series of **bricks** *(Another item you'd likely find lying about.)* and hey presto - a *6 cardboard/hardboard* ramp!

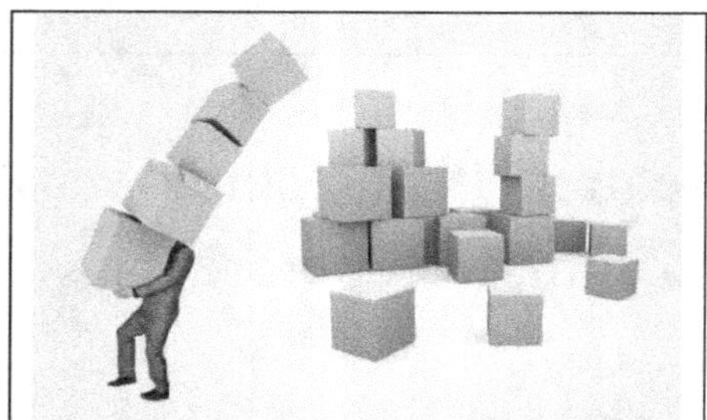  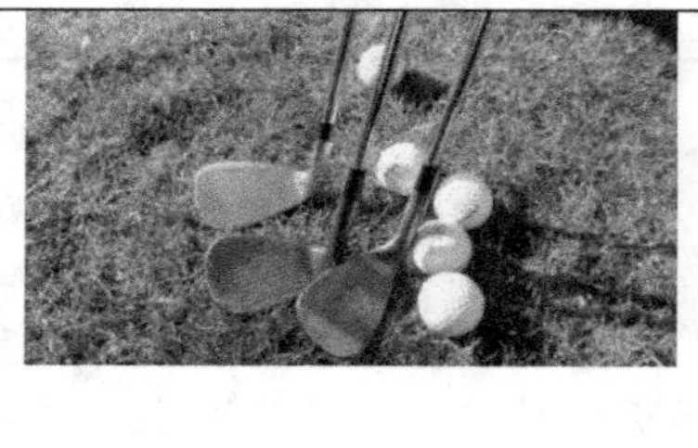

The picture earlier, of the OAP, is most appropriate as the Golfing Aficionado Grand-Parent(s) can take part in this also – Hoorah! (And try to beat their younger opponents!)

It can get really competitive when all are playing the same hole together – especially if there is no rule against your hitting your opponent's ball out of the way with your shot! Too Evil?

OFF YOU GO TRY ME

A5iii) The Obstacle Course is made of the same materials as the Golf Course, but the handicapping can be uniquely different from that of a standard Golf Game.

If Dad etc is/are too good with bats/clubs so little Johnny/Jenny are getting fed up you have two options:

1. A time penalty, or
2. A bat penalty – simply put, give Dad + any other of the best a broom right way up, to steer their ball! (The taller the bristles the better!

The end of the obstacle course is either hitting a specific object, or getting your ball between two specific sticks

OFF YOU GO TRY ME

WHEELIE BIN CHIPS OFF THE OLD BLOCK:

A6 Like A1 above, but with an additional Dad v Son skill factor.

So, it is all from 1, minus the paddling pool, substituted by the wheelie bin, suitably, lined *23* for health's sake + the addition of *Footballs, 10* .

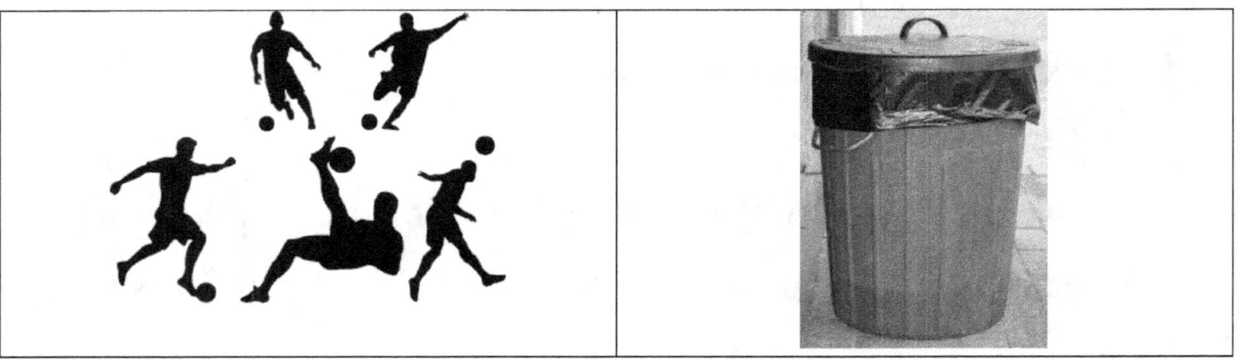

i) Yes this is the dry version, but, the bin will provide the football challenge, as whoever thinks they are the best: from whatever distance, each tries to chip the ball into the bin!

ii) Perhaps, set up 2, having two playing at once and see who can do it first, within a reasonable time limit. And here those Yankee Lady World Champion Footballers can show their male counterparts what they are made of!

Power to the Female?

PS For those who play you can substitute your Rugby Ball!

But, really, the Wheelie Bins are a great source of competitive inter-family/friends challenges#.

And here are some more:

<u>WHEELIE BIN ADAPTATIONS:</u>

And here are some more:

iii) Your golf challenge could incorporate them as special hazards to get your ball around, or through.

Use this also as another target to throw your tennis ball between.

If placed wide enough, from a certain distance: the closer for the less able.

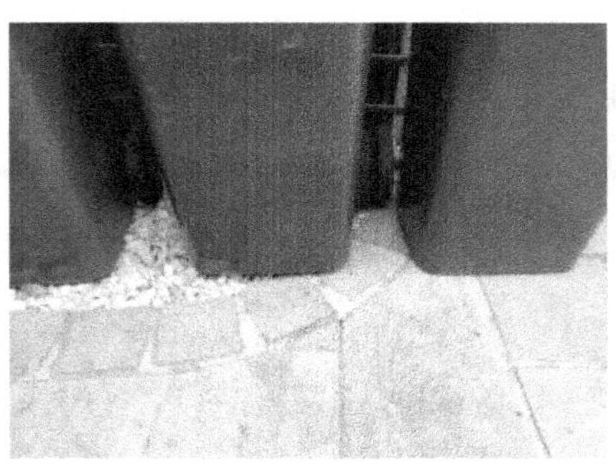

↓

iv) The bins when placed wheels side-by-side *22a*, with the wheels **<u>away from you</u>**, you will notice a natural gap before you: use as a golf hole, at the end of your course (rule example, one stroke penalty if you miss altogether, or get in an impossible position, then in both instances have a designated spot where balls are repositioned!).

Easy? Well, then have the bins around the corner, facing away (A dirty dog leg if ever there was one!) to make it more difficult?

v) 22 **<u>Set them</u>** up now in a row, lids flipped over out of the way, and the next throwing-accurately challenge can be played from whichever distance is agreed upon *(With no football in sight!)*.

Then just see how many times (out of 10) one can throw the tennis ball into the bin.

Or

How many times (out of 10) one can, using cricket bat/tennis racquet /badminton racquet loop/hit/throw the tennis ball/shuttle over/into the bin. (Even using a Lacrosse Stick + Ball?)

Make it more difficult?

vi) Here it might be oddly funnily & ever so slightly dangerous for the one adjacent the Bin(s), likely 2 the maximum, unless you can make the lids stand up on their own! –

Turn the Bins around so the lid is up, obstructing your view of the hole then recommence your attempts above!

But here a looping trajectory is paramount!

So it's the badminton Gear Only!

Although, remember be careful with your aim >>>
– so best do it one person at a time, or Dad might get a sore head
– shuttlecock bottoms are much harder than your/his head first imagined!

OFF YOU GO TRY ME

WATER PISTOL/MARBLE TARGET MIXES:

A7a *I purposely omitted them 21, Marbles from A6vi) above for obvious safety reasons: shuttlecock bottoms have nothing on a marble or two striking your head, thrown from a distance away!*

We, who had nothing, those bygone years, could just about afford a bag of marbles to play with them on the street pavements, or back yards and so with them in mind we need the following:

21, Marbles, 5a & b, Used Plastic Bottles, 6, Ramp 4, Buckets 20, Water pistols, 17 Cricket =the stumps only.

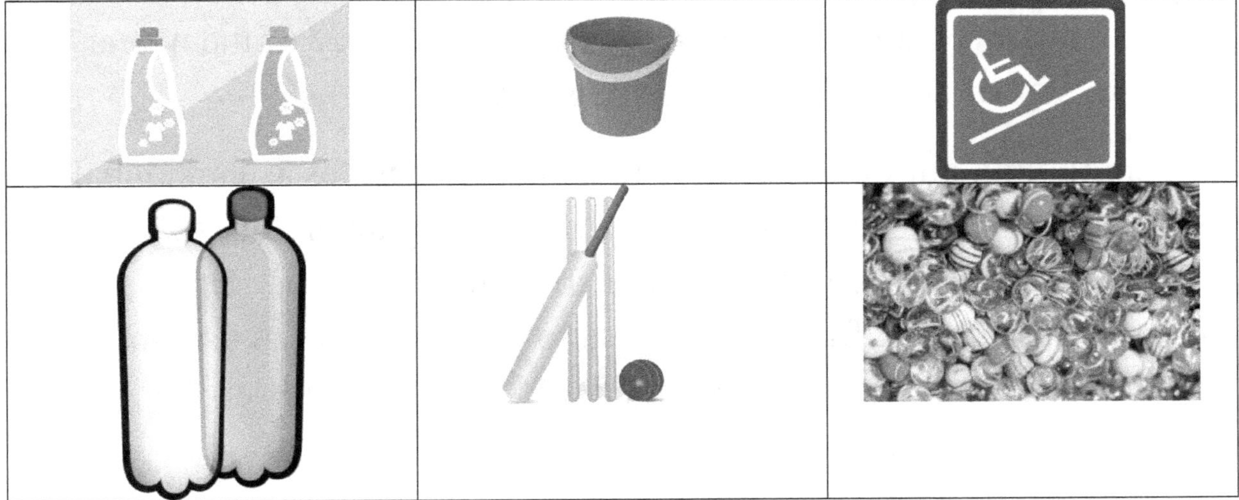

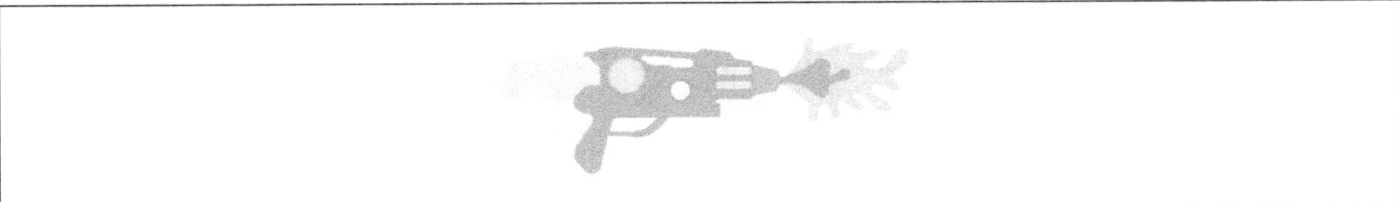

i) This might need some supervision in case it gets slightly out of hand – so only allow 10 marbles at a time then refresh when used up.

This is so simple, in its simplicity, you can just see how many of yours you can toss into that half-filled bucket – the most = the winner.

The reason there is water in the bucket, is safety first again, just in case one marble breaks another inside.

However, because marbles were a worthy/bartering commodity, we used to adapt the game, as we had no goodie rewards coming our way, we added this specific rule: he/she who tosses their marble into the bucket first, picks up/wins those which missed their target.

But, here, at the end of the game the marble = sweets.

It was a copy of the game we played flicking cards against a wall trying to knock those, which were originally stood up to knock over!

Or, you also won all if one of your cards covered any of them near the wall – a sort of double chance flicking game!

So, continuing our outdoor pursuit: using our marbles as cannonballs, we can use the plastic bottles and cartons (Flat side on top, so sweet falls off easier!) as targets, scattered about in front of us. This will be of particular interest for those parents to get their boys to use up all that pent up aggression want so badly to knock the objects over – <u>underarm always AND always in turn</u>!

And ensure something soft behind the targets to soften the force of the marble – If brickwork then use the cardboard to cushion the impact and this will also guarantee the marble doesn't crack/chip etc on impact.

Here the sweet giving is not necessary as they are placed upon the cartons and bottle tops! You win what you knock over.

BUT - Here, handle with care – <u>when the sweet drops stop the game</u> and hand the sweet to the person who knocked it over.

Hello Humble Used Loo Roll:

Perhaps for the toddler types we can tone it down a few notches and introduce our soft, easy to knock over _humble_ used toilet rolls – here their adaption _sets them above_ so many others, because they are hollow and so you can stand them on their end and hide the sweet inside.

You can make it more entertaining by having different numbers of small sweets hidden inside – then it's a bit of pot luck who wins more.

There again to prevent disappointed tears always ensure even the losers win something – but they need be taught you cannot always be the winner – it's just a fact of life they need be taught before they meet their _'real world opponents!'_

_ii)_ To make it harder for likely the older male element, use cricket stamps knocked into the earth and the sweet(s) balanced on the hollow, in line with you and not at 90 degrees, where the stumps usually slot in.

    Then, tennis balls are thrown at the sweet carrying stumps.

For these types of throwing games, the _only_ caveat is that it helps to have a wall at the end to bounce back against – so two chances to hit your target.

And, if there is one, then, once again those delivery cardboard boxes come in handy – perhaps flattened out first, and lain against the brickwork! (Not broken/torn apart as they always can/will come in useful at other times.) Better still if the cardboard forms a ramp, down which the balls can roll back down?

iii) Enough throwing, then here we can introduce the water pistol filled from our pool reservoir with its water being the wet bullet trying to shoot down their prize! The shooting ends when all the sweets are downed!

Likely the fun will be when the guns start running out, with the accompanying frenzy to refill them before the opponent guns down the remaining sweet(s)!

If you gauge the distance too far at first, then always feel free to foreshorten it to avoid child frustration!

You can adapt this game substituting the marble for the sweet and the marbles won are exchanged for sweets at the end.

OFF YOU GO TRY ME

MARBLE RAMPING IT UP & DOWN:

A7b 5, Used Plastic Bottles 21, Marbles 6 Ramp= (cardboard)

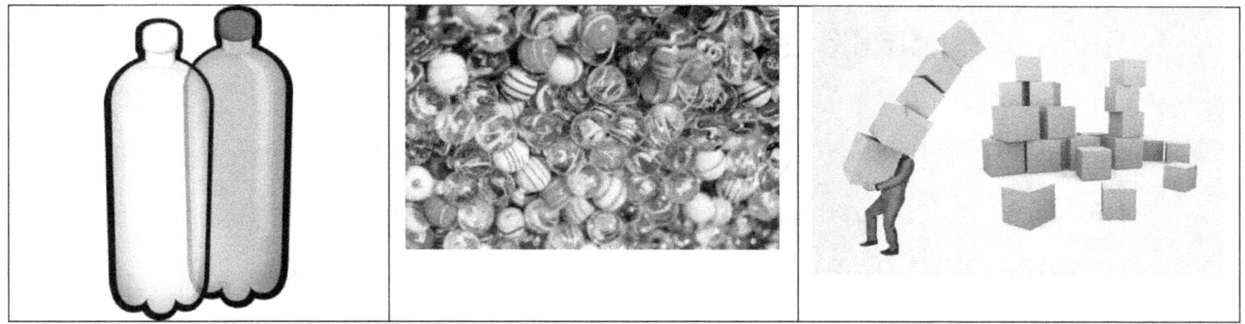

<u>You'll need a bit of skill here and perhaps Dad should go first?</u>

i This will work on paving, rather than grass, so no need for having to hammer home the cricket stumps. Actually, you'll just need 2 old plastic bottles standing upright next to each other, say a foot apart and about a couple of metres from you, to either the left or right – it is quite immaterial. But what is most important is that you are along from AND in line with the bottles – even place an old **brick** or two between you both...

ii The object of the game is to roll the marbles between the bottles and points = sweets. But how can you if you are in line with the bottles? And, not forgetting, that obstructing **brick** in your line of fire!

iii So the ingenious amongst your family, utilising that spare cardboard, need build a ramp down from you; up another ramp just to the side of you from which the marble rolls/is directed towards its/between the bottles target, thus the obstructing brick is negated – Understand?

iv Your ramp down will be in the form of a gully – made by folding in half the cardboard you hold and then easier to point.

v Be prepared for it not to work the first couple of times, as you have to make sure the marble is able to have a smooth run – one problem will be making sure there is no obstructing gap between the two ramps!

vi Obviously, after all that effort, Dad goes first to show how easy it is/isn't?

OFF YOU GO TRY ME

<u>BE CAREFUL DARTING:</u>

A8 Has a twist to a certain skilful, UK dominated game:

Grass Darts!

And so, from the list above, let's hope you have the following:

1. *18, Dart board + Darts 19, 25 Delivery/Packing Boxes*

Recalling ↑ Way Back OUCH!

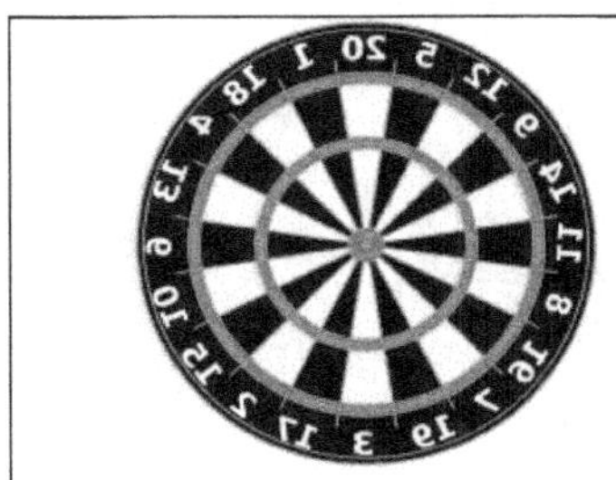 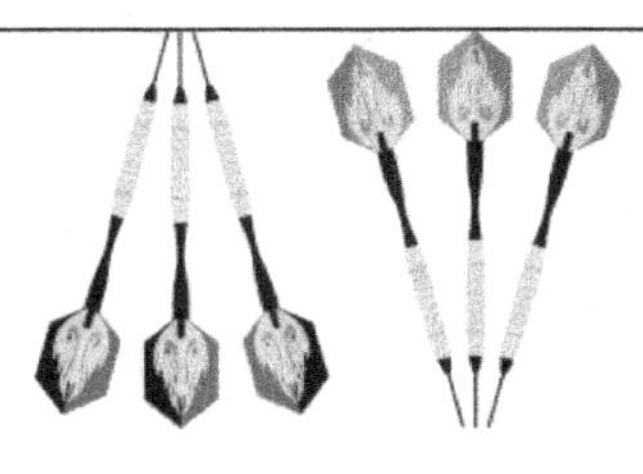 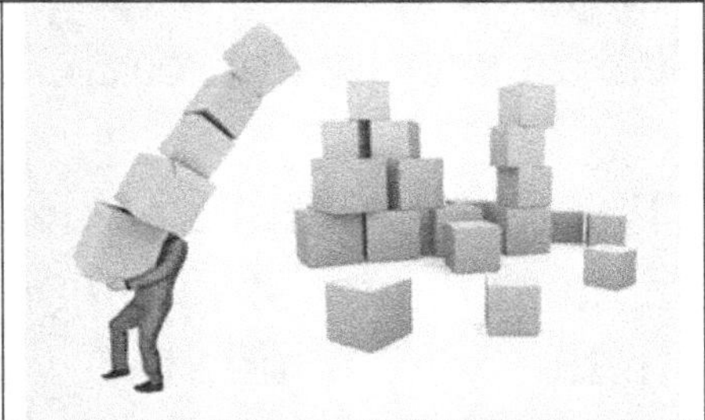

<u>Here follows a Parental Warning ></u>

In that long forgotten, golden era of my youth, we, as kids, were left very much to our own devices to wander and play as we felt we wanted to: so we played football in the streets; disappeared along train lines playing dodge; knocking on doors and running away...And so it will come as no surprise as this is something you'd never allow in your child's household. We used to throw the dart high in the air and a colleague *(Always a silly boy, not a sensible girl in sight!)* **would hold the dartboard in front of him trying to catch the dart on the board.**
Yes, you're right one was not that well-co-ordinated and so his wrist was the recipient of the darts sharp point.
But, hey, those were the days; the simple thing to do was just pull it out – strangely <u>*not much blood*</u> GUSHED from the wound.

i) Set the board on the ground/grass at your prescribed distance from the thrower (shorter for the less capable) everyone stand clear and hey presto TOSS and hope your total darts score is the winning one!

ii) Or you could try Blind-Fold darts! Allow the thrower one last look before you mask him/her then laugh at the horrible efforts – a sort of play on pin the donkey. BUT make sure you are behind the thrower!
iii) There again, you could expand upon this by using your cardboard *25,* – the one piece you cut into many.
Sprinkle them in a loose circular cluster front of the shooter with various scores on each.
<u>Then, it's hit and hope!</u>
The reason for the tighter cluster circle is that an arbitrary throw has a better chance of hitting something!
In this way it aids the youngest/much older/less adept.

OFF YOU GO TRY ME

<u>It might be suggested with the balloons & darts to hand, one could be target practice for the other.</u> **<u>My one & only warning would be darts do bounce of in all directions if they don't stick to the balloon. So, stick to avoiding this variation!</u>**

<u>Anyhow, I have less dangerous wet usage for the balloons!</u>

Hey, what about the Washing Line(s)?

<u>BALLOON/BIN LINERS PARTY TIME:</u>

A9a And so, from the list above, let's hope you have the following:
22 + 23(liners), 24 Balloons.

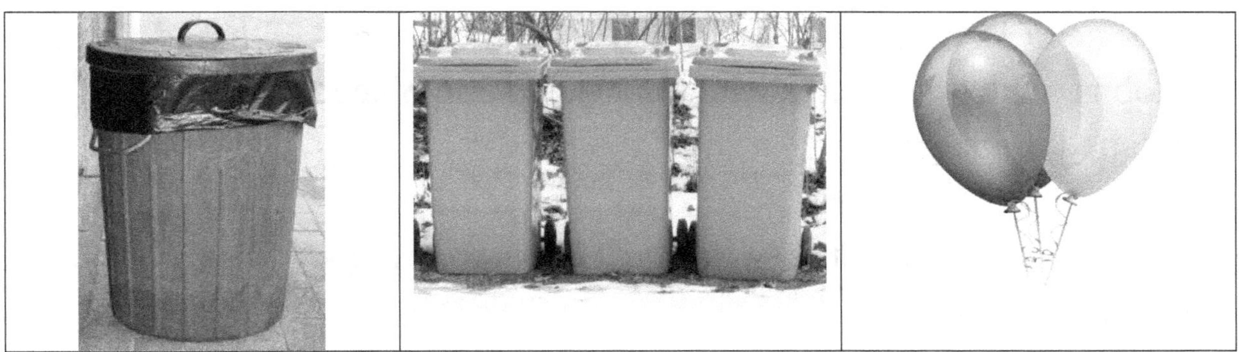

The usual convention at birthday parties is for one, they all seem to be organised by some outsider.

But, and it is a Big Potentially Financial Big But, we all cannot for out £250 for a Bouncy Castle, or paid group attendance in an adventure playground complete with slides/maze/climbing frames etc.

So, if it is at your place with a select half a dozen or so invitees for your child, this will do admirably for what we have in mind.

The usual convention a birthday parties is for one, they all seem to give out their goodie bags, as people begin to leave.

But, and it is a Big Audience Surprising Big But, what if the collecting Mums have to sit, wait & watch what unfolds before their eyes – something completely unexpected?

And so enter our *22s, & 24s.* But, not another Easter Egg Hunt, more based on my/an Xmas Present Trail Variation which follows this one.

We are hunting for a Key Clue to where the Goodie Bags have been stashed – here the age group must be of reading capability, especially the birthday girl/boy.

Apologies here as there is a little bit of effort: for say 20 balloons, you'll need 18 bogus notes and two special ones, placed in individual balloons, which you then need to blow up and place in loosely selotaped bin bags.

The bogus notes will just say *I don't know where the goodie bags are!* The other two will say:
 *(1) **What goes on a washing line and holds the clothes up?***
*(2) **In what bag are they kept?***

The instruction you give them is to find the 2 bags with clues as to the whereabouts of the goodie bags.

To make it easier to distinguish the special clues, is to write them out in bold red with the others being in plain black/blue.

So, the whole party are made to go into the garden outside and told that there is a clue or two in the balloons contained in the Bin Bags hanging from (<u>not tied to</u>) shrubs/trees, prepared by you just beforehand. Even the washing line with a bag (Clue) pegged to it, which has/had its play here too earlier?

So, all the participants are told to empty the bags & grab the balloons and burst them to find/read the note inside.

The mothers looking on will see the mad noisy scramble for the clues in the balloons and jump at the incessant popping of bursting balloons.

Now the important part of the puzzle hoping that the 2 clues are found, but not the answer – here you come in, whatever the result.

It is common in gardens to have the peg bag outside hanging from the line, or an outside hook, but so usually behind the back door, out of sight when it is opened. If not, try to arrange a similar scene.

Then, if all are stumped reveal the peg bag as the answer and get birthday boy/girl to get it down and find the answer envelope – this again prewritten by you:

"The key you want was hanging behind me – it will open the garage (or shed door whichever) where your goodie bags are hidden [M] – one for each of you!"

[M] Make it easy by having the Bag just inside the locked door...

The last hurdle for the hungry party people is for your special party girl/boy to find the key within the SIX (or so) you have on the key chain/ring, which opens the lock (padlock in my case).

OFF YOU GO TRY ME

<u>KIDS TARGETED/BAGGED PRIZE MIXES:</u>

Here is a *derivatory* twist of the above/aforementioned – I hope you like it and try it...

A9b Another kiddies' game idea, which would distract them from annoying all, but a couple * + Daddy &/or Mummy...

Say there were two nippers, who needed stimulating and exciting...

1. You've just come back from holiday, or are celebrating something special where presents might be the order of the day.
2. But, and it is a Big But (to stretch time out) they must be distributed <u>one at a time</u>.
3. Let the kids know that <u>their</u> individual special gifts are <u>in the garage</u>, shed etc. and the keys are in one of the bags outside.
4. Let them view you hanging the bags (plastic/whatever is handy) outside – best to be <u>at the end of the garden</u> **
5. There are two children, then, you need at least 4, or 6, present bags, so each can deal with 2, or 3, (to avoid the usual he/she has got more than me).
6. But, and it is an even Bigger But, so the presents are in tied bags hanging from trees etc in the garden outside, which must be taken down one at a time and <u>brought back singly for inspection</u>.
7. As the bags can only be brought back one at a time, the next child cannot start until the full contents of the previous bag have been revealed and distributed
8. But, and it is another similar Big But (to stretch time out), the presents are hung far too high for the kids so each must go with <u>your</u> allocated adult each (usually one for each sex - ie 2* in total) to help them bring them back.
9. They must be brought back to one of their parents to untie and distribute.

10.   It will be discovered by the kids that the keys are not in any of the bags they brought back, just some minor sweets (or whatever you decide) – So?

11.   There is another bag (as the game above), which most people would have forgotten about, and this is where the layout of most houses is important that the washing line and peg bag are usually adjacent to the back door and as it opens it hides this area so keep it in this position throughout (And this is where you kept the 2 nominated adults (2 *) in the loop so as not to spoil the future surprise) Hence the hiding of the bags at the opposite end** to distract the kids eyes/thoughts!

12.   So? If the real deal peg bag is not picked, then it is a case of bringing the kids back inside and telling them that the bag they seek is still outside. Tell them the Adults will help.

13.   So? Then send the kids out & as they go searching, the adults inside via the open back door still concealing the peg bag, do the shouting out a bit of _hot and cold_ to assist in the final bag search.

14.   When they find it and the keys inside – Success will come although the adult couple * might need to help as some are hooked quite high up.

15.   But, and it is yet another Big But, it is not the end of things.

16.   The bag contains a large bunch of keys and it is then up to the usually older infant to try to ascertain (by trial and error) which is the right key - Success will come, although the adult couple * might need to help.

OFF YOU GO TRY ME

SPARE BOX IMAGINATION TARGETED:

We cannot always guarantee sunshine each day – rain does come
always uninvited, but that is not something which should spoil the
younger kids fun time.
Yes, there is always the Computer etc...
But, let's still be creative/imaginative and Hey presto the larger
Cardboard Boxes will come into their element and won't be too
broken up so can be later used for something else.

Indoor Interlude:- *25, Delivery/Packing Boxes +*
31= roll of tape & scissors. (And Patience!)

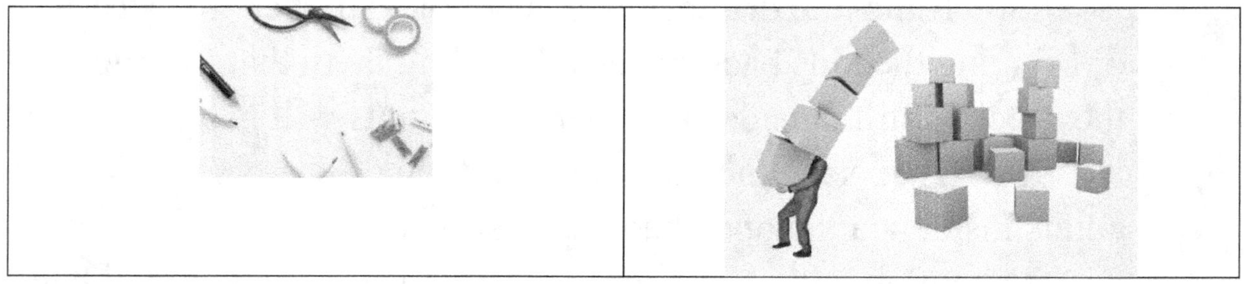

So, Granddaddy, Daddy, Big Brother the youngsters need you help
and undivided attention – Ah! They said please, so how can you
refuse!
Build me/us a Doll's House, with windows and doors so I can look
inside!
Build me/us our own Card-Board House so we disappear/hide inside!
So, Granddaddy, Daddy, Big Brother, do you think you are up to it?
The youngsters will help you by cutting the Tape!

There again, as Dad can keep them occupied with his *'building'*
skills? Did he remember that Doll's Houses open out in two halves,
sideways towards you?

And, as a Kid's House, then the opening is at one end or the other –
and, be careful, as that taped roof structure will be affected by it?
Mummy has it easy: "Kids, would you like the bake a cake with me?"
I'll let you lick the spatula/spoon dry!

<u>**Indoor Interlude (2):-**</u> *25, Delivery/Packing Boxes +*

31= roll of tape & scissors. (And Even More Patience!)

Here the difficulty rating is on the up!

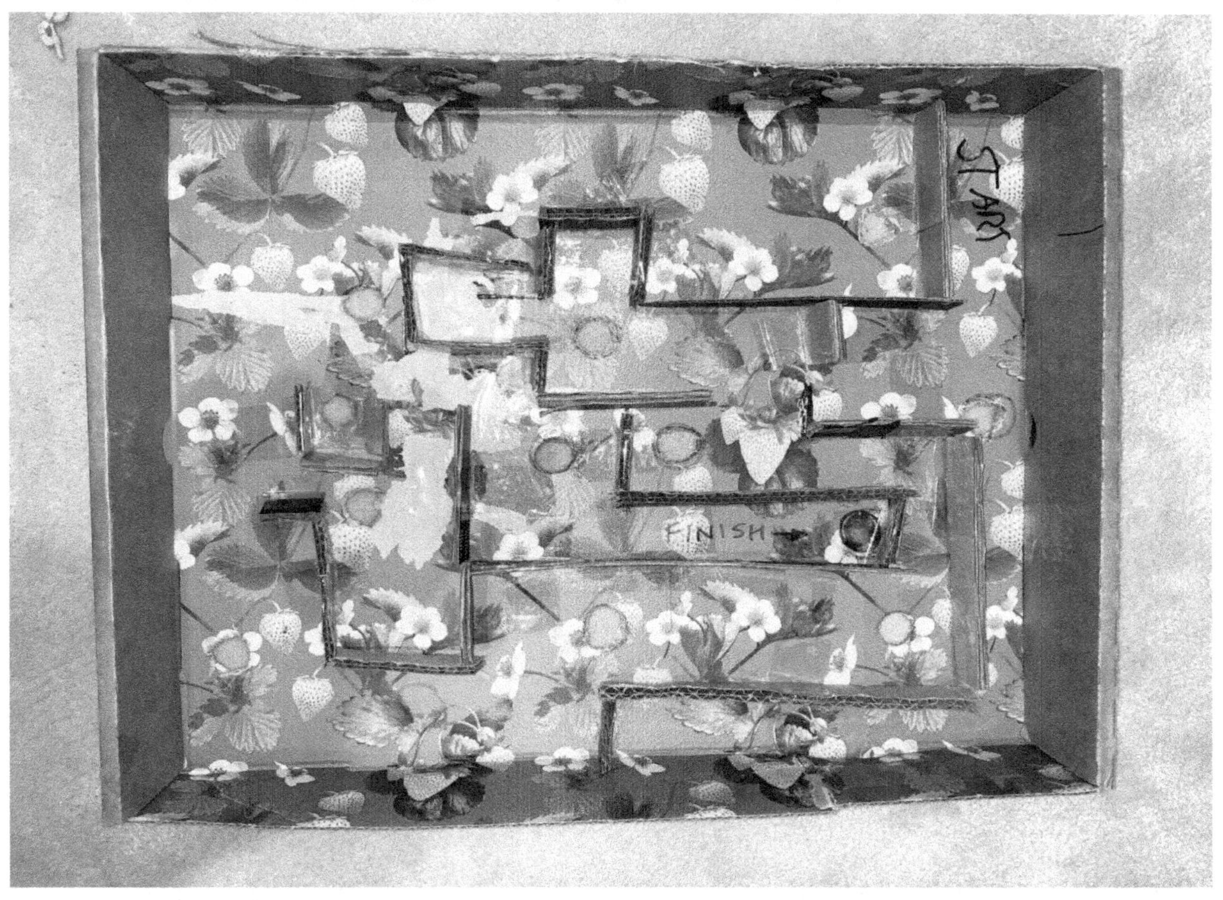

↑(The Example Above was made by an 8 year old!)↑

Build your own Marble *Holed* Maze – so many designs to choose from!

https://www.google.com/search?source=univ&tbm=isch&q=marble +maze&client=firefox-b-d&sa=X&ved=2ahUKEwi50a3NofLpAhWAQxUIHZnBDfQQsAR6BA gBEAE

OFF YOU GO TRY ME

INDOOR COURSE MANAGEMENT:

From Outdoors to Indoors – in Stages!

Hey, yes you can play the golf game(s) on paving, but, "Where's the hole?" you cry: your humble delivery cardboard box comes into its own again, to the rescue.

Take it apart gently to its flat state and you will discover if you lay it down face up, it naturally is raised off the ground.

You will also notice all four flaps are off the ground, also.
So, simply cut your hole in the middle and you have a natural incline to the hole area – if you get your hole in _'won'_ is another matter!

So with that outdoor solution in mind it is starting to rain – no worries!

How you thought you can easily adapt the aforementioned, inside.

First, let us not forget, the equipment for outdoors might be too _'furniture'_ dangerous for the indoors – so adapt softer!

That sorted, it's back to our humble cardboard: if you have a large enough room inside, then you can attack your 'golf-hole' area from 4 sides, just as you could outside.

But, so many might not have such an indoor open space: there is always the Hall!

Adapt your cardboard ramp to long-ways, with the sides up: they might not be in use, but it is best not to cut up a perfectly usable ex-box – it might be needed again in its intact state.

With this set up you can have one (set) of players at both ends!

But, there is another permutation.

Here, all play from one end: If you raise the lengthways side, furthest from you, up against the door, with the sides up also, you have a natural ramp system and possibly a second opportunity to score on the way back!

OFF YOU GO TRY ME

From a Summer Sport to a Winter Adapted One

Indoor/Outdoor Plastic Slalom:

- *Here lay out your plastic bottle course (washing up liquid/shower/softener – the availability is endless, but not rectangular items like washing machine pod containers as these are not knock <u>overable</u>!*
- *Get the kids to do individual timed runs in & out of the bottle course.*
- *Or if you have the space one v one with 2 identical courses prepared.*
- *Use a tennis ball as the item then need negotiate the course.*
- *It can be propelled by feet/hockey stick/or whatever is appropriately to hand – outdoors one can use a foot/football combination as space would presumably allow this.*
- *If a bottle is knocked over then the participant must put it back on its allotted spot before continuing.*
- *As a bit of mischief, if possible, put a sweet on top of selected bottles and this will ensure no mad rushing as it would be a case of knock-it-off at your peril as it would be handed to your opponent! Although it is yours if you win the round!*

Now (Un)Controlled Bouncing Chaos!

Part 1: Parents will notice their offspring from an early age will have a fascination with the staircase.

So, why not let them have free rein? – Just make sure any prized breakables are not in their '*firing*' line!

To help in that respect, make sure your ball is of the softer side.

Yes, smaller might be seem totally sensible, but not that monstrous bouncing kind – havoc is guaranteed, unless well controlled, as perhaps, this example?

To improve their co-ordination, have one infant set the ball in motion from the top of the stairs and see if the one at the bottom can (ultimately) catch it?

Knowing its capability, the child might catch it on the way back rebounded from the front door?

A word of warning: Don't have more than one at the bottom catching, as it is likely a bigger child will invariably knock the smaller over!

Now (Un)Controlled Bouncing Chaos!

Part 2a: So, that mini '*extreme*' bouncer might be too uncontrollable, so it's back to basics – Tennis Balls & Co!

These however do not lend themselves successfully to the catching game above.

So, what now?

Well, if you have a few and those left over washing up bottles, softener bottles & empty cans, then here they will come into their element.

Place them indiscriminately down the steps (at least 6 away) for the person on the top to roll balls down, hoping to knock them over – most wins!

So, kids, are you in line at the top there?

Or, have one at the top playing and another at the bottom collecting the balls and objects knocked over – keeping score too, as we must not forget the object of the game – winning (sweets?) or some other goodie dangled before them – your choice.

By the way scoring is not that easy!

OFF YOU GO TRY ME

Now (Un)Controlled *Marble* Bouncing Chaos!

Part 2b

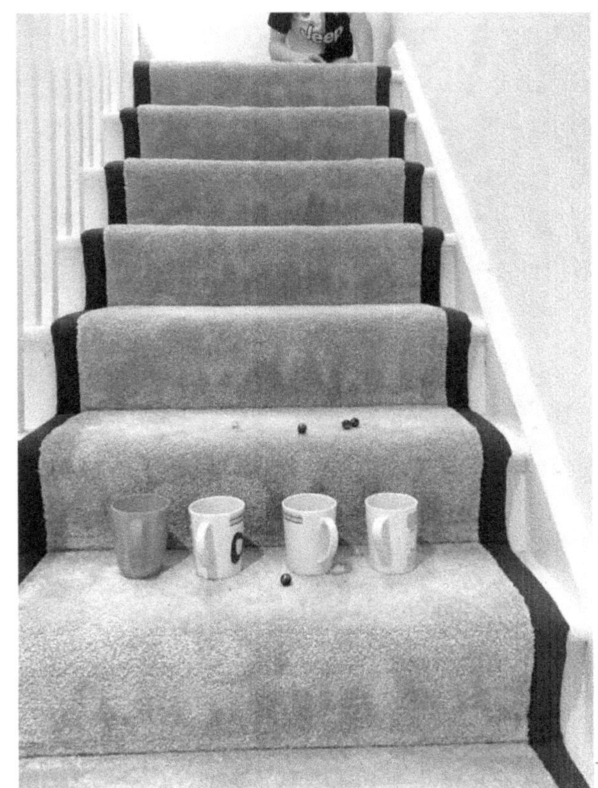

I think it speaks for itself: Use marbles instead of balls and see how many the child(ren) can direct into the plastic mugs/cups/beakers. Or just use your kitchen mugs, but not glass of any kind, as it might shatter.

Your course can be as many steps as you wish!

One additional word of care is to make sure you know how many marbles you started with and that you have <u>rounded them all up</u>: you don't want anybody slipping over them later on!

OFF YOU GO TRY ME

Now (Un)Controlled Bouncing Golfing Chaos!
Part 3: You can increase this adaptation
Again soft balls & clubs, if possible.

Around your ground floor rooms, you can arrange for an object to be a substitute hole, and the kids/adults must manoeuvre their ball to be in a position to knock it over.
The blessing here is that furniture can be a natural hazard – hoping that it is not too hazardous for any ornaments standing around in their mis-directed way!
But, like before the staircase above, it can be brought into the kid's mind mix, as the tee off is at the top of the stairs!
It just adds a different element to the game.

If you have a second staircase, well, the '*exciting*' better
So, with a complete melding, you can arrange a household course as follows:
  i.   Down staircase, into a designated room *(keep the adjoining doors closed)*; if a bedroom, then you have the largest natural hazard, so put your pin object around the other side.
  ii. Yes, some beds might be well above the ground, but just a hint of what fun might happen if the child tries for a shot underneath! Yes, the ball only reaches halfway & runs out of reach.

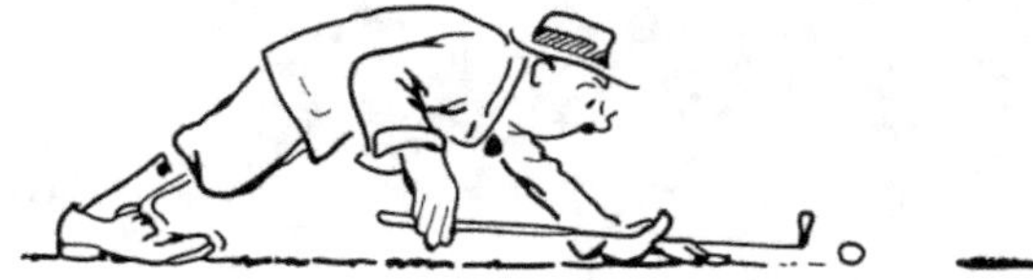

  iii. Remember Old grandad?
  iv. Here their adaptability might come into play: they, either crawl beneath and push, or, if they cannot get properly beneath the

bed, they'll have to use that specialist Broom Handle Club? So, keep it handy?

    v.   Then, it's down to the lounge etc.

    vi.   Your course will obviously consist of all available rooms.

OFF YOU GO TRY ME

Now (Un)Controlled Bouncing Footballing Chaos!

Part 4: Just the kicking version of the above for those budding World Cup Stars, or think they are?

- Again, the ball is small/soft;
- The blessing is that there are no clubs swinging about around the furniture!
- The kicking need not be hard in view of the confined spaces;
- Here the child's ability to direct the ball where he/she wants it to go is sorely tested;
- Down the stairs is not always achieved with just one kick – if their ball gets stuck up against anything, allow the child to move it a few inches away, so he/she can place their kicking foot behind!
- Needless to say, no flashy lobs, one never knows where they may end up – the TV screen is no match, is one to be avoided example!
- Like above, one think paramount, the number of tries must be strictly monitored/counted – especially where the ball gets stuck under the child's slipper – Is that a shot?
- Dad would be in charge so what could go wrong?

OFF YOU GO TRY ME

Now (Un)Controlled Bouncing Balloon Chaos!

Part 5: Balloons Games outside are sorely trying if the Wind takes control of their flight.
But, inside the control is all yours, or so you lead the kids to believe: they'll find out their control is so limited!

- You'll also need something with a large opening like your humble bin, or laundry basket, but try and ensure your balloon is small enough to fit the available opening.
- From varying distances see how many hits the child takes to direct his/her balloon from the start to the finish ...
- The finish is getting the balloon inside the bin/basket.
- It takes much longer than they/you would imagine!
- One proviso – they get a penalty stroke every time the balloon hits the floor.
- Only one hand can be used, the other kept behind their back!
- One can place obstacles in the way, but this is not like the golf game above, so have regard to the safety first factor: as a principle, I'd avoid such things.
- If you have say four contestants, you can arrange them in 6 different pairings: AB, AC, AD, BC, BD, CD
- So there is no Bias, as each will be paired with both the best & the worst!
- Here the Lowest Accumulative Score wins
- One piece of advice: blow the balloons up well, the less pumped up, the quicker they fall!

OFF YOU GO TRY ME

Now (Un)Controlled Volleyball Balloon Chaos!

Part 6: Again the critical factor is your home space in your corridor?

If you have sufficient free space, here is one for the more/most

energetic, as they will slowly but surely discover, scoring is nigh

impossible, as it depends on the number of times you can handle the

balloon, which here should be _on the smaller size_.

- Volleyball, if memory serves, allows 3 hits.
- Employ this for the game initially,
- You might find 2 is sufficient later to make it easier to score!
- Always initially place the younger child with his/her back to the door – this makes sure the elder has more space to cover!
- So in the corridor that humble badminton net will be useful.
- Roll up the ends to suit the width of the corridor
- Tie these up with humble cotton thread
- It is essential you use something which will break under strain: you don't want the dado rail getting yanked from the wall?!
- Drawing Pin the cotton ends to each side of the dado rail above;
- The pinning should be hard, but Let it hang at whichever level suits the two contestants
- Well above head height the best to avoid too many easy smashes
- So off you go.
- The only proviso here is that this is mainly for the much younger element to spend time hitting away AND NOT for the Senior School Attendee – send these to the Beach!

OFF YOU GO TRY ME

OUTDOOR LINE PRIZE MANAGEMENT:

AND NOW IS THE WASHING LINE'S TURN!

A10 You can make your children a simple obstacle course should the fancy take you, but why risk a tripping/slipping injury amongst all the mayhem.

- You could organise party races where for instance two teams compete to bring balls form from bucket at the far end of the garden, to another back with you, but why put yourself within a dispute spot, or find your special party girl/boy upset at losing the race(s) claiming their ball was in first but the bucket fell over etc...

- Hence, the idea to involve all in a common pursuit goal, after possibly having been kept inside for other types of less demanding fun/video viewing/other indoor party games like pass the parcel/musical chairs, to name a few.

- So, this washing line (or large ball of string) will be a special one, used in two ways: the group and/or individual, not unlike the key chase above.

- Again preparation is the _key_ (_sorry_) and the longer the line the better #; the supervisory/help aspect, as it arises. (# _So, if not, just try to have two at your disposal_)(Or start with the ball of string and have its end attached to that of the washing line!).

OFF YOU GO TRY ME

A10i) The Group: If we have six children participating we need six goodie bags numbered 1 to 6: one being the first to be claimed.

Before the start each child draws a number, so Number 1 goes first.

But, for the child to claim his/her prize he/she needs to unravel, unwind their part of the line/rope maze.

Why unravel? Because you have spent time winding your line/rope all around the garden, inside & round shrubs/trees, in and out of garden furniture, even through the hole at the top of closed padlocks; plant supports and the like, anything which would pose as an obstacle – you get my drift. You'll also be aware which plants to avoid as we don't want your prize specimen being torn apart, or little Johnny/Jenny getting cut up by one of your prickly Rose Bushes!

So, <u>you start at the end</u> where you leave No6, then ravel some until you come to No5 and so on, until, some way off the beginning, where you attach No1.

Attach?

At each goodie bag retrieval stage tie the two side handles around the line/rope, tight enough so it won't easily come loose, but so strong enough that it poses some effort from the child getting it to slide off.

When child No1 gets his/her prize and before starting to start chewing etc, he/she hands over the rope to No2 and so it goes on.

It is up to you if all the bags contain the same sweets – if not I'm sure the kids might try to swap? Never know?

OFF YOU GO TRY ME

A10ii) + *22* Now the line/rope is unravelled, tie a slip knot at both ends; put a stake next to you (start & finish area). The stake is critical as you need it to be well seated in the earth but not pointed at the upright end as we don't want faces/eyes poked.

As you have a slip knot you can use a broom, placing the pointed end in the earth **, brush end on top #: this also tests the child's hopefully prior awareness slip knots can expand, although all they might know from this initially is that it also tightens! But not too hard, we hope? ##

(** *If you have one then the parasol base of your garden table umbrella?*)

(Additional word of warning/advice this is a game for the lawn rather than paving as kids do fall over and the grass is so forgiving in comparison:
But it is up to the Host/Organiser!)

Now you have the option of individuals, or teams – remembering there is always a sweet prize for both winners & losers, only that the winners get a little more!

It is simple in its ingenuity as the rope is rolled up before each round; one slip knot is placed fully over the stake # so that it drops to floor level and tightened in situ.

The other loop is around the child's wrist (*Or waist*) ##.

If we play singly and presumably it is a *'fastest'* time wins race, then the participant must undo the slip knot from his/her wrist/waist and extend it so it can go over the brush/stake and the timing watch is stopped when the rope hits the floor.

But now we must consider the *22* Wheelie Bin(s) Role: either one just far away so there is enough spare line/rope to unravel and flip over the upright broom/brush/stake; or if we use more than one Bin make sure you allow for those awkward corners.

- Knowing how excited some children can get and lose all sense of logic, brief them beforehand that the line can get stuck at the most inopportune moment and they will be held back: tugging might only exacerbate the situation, especially if rooted under the Bin Wheel. So, it is best they focus/calm down and go back to where it is stuck and sort it.
- If you use more than one Bin to manoeuvre about, then there are bound to be a few more Wheelie snags!
- The other aspect is that the Child only focuses on the end in his/her hand and becomes unaware of mounting snags as not all the rope gets pulled completely past each possible snagging area and it is when they are yards short at the end do they realise that they need return to the problem area(s) and get the rest of the slack they need to flip the slip knot over your chosen stake <> broom/brush/umbrella stand head!

OFF YOU GO TRY ME

A10iii) With teams, the only rule addition is that after the slip knot is put over the broom head AND touches the ground the runner must take his/her seat and then the next can start, retracing their games partner's steps#.

Here, a minor complication that you avoid: make the route complicated and confusion will ensue, unless you want it to – you can always use an aid/something to map out the route for the kids (Chalk anyone?) (Pieces of cardboard stuck to the floor with arrows written on them).

 # I would suggest the second/subsequent ones (back & forwards) should only have to run around the Bin furthest away, rather than the convoluted route the first runner had to encounter. It will be hard enough dragging the rope around behind them!

Best accumulative time wins twice as many sweet as the runners up – <u>Remember losers never go empty handed!</u>

And so if you wish to get involved No30 comes into play as all can participate – Hurry up Grandad/Grandma!   ↓↓ *Helping Hand...*

<u>**No30 = The Family – no matter how good or bad at it??**</u>

<u>**Although, most likely, the kids will not have such patience!**</u>

....

OFF YOU GO TRY ME

OUTDOOR/INDOOR CARD MANIPILATION:

Continuing with the Whole Family Theme –No30 – Here is one which is normally played indoors, but is just as much fun, perhaps more, when outside – but strong winds would deter you, for the obvious fly away reason!

A11 <u>CARD PAIRS</u>:-

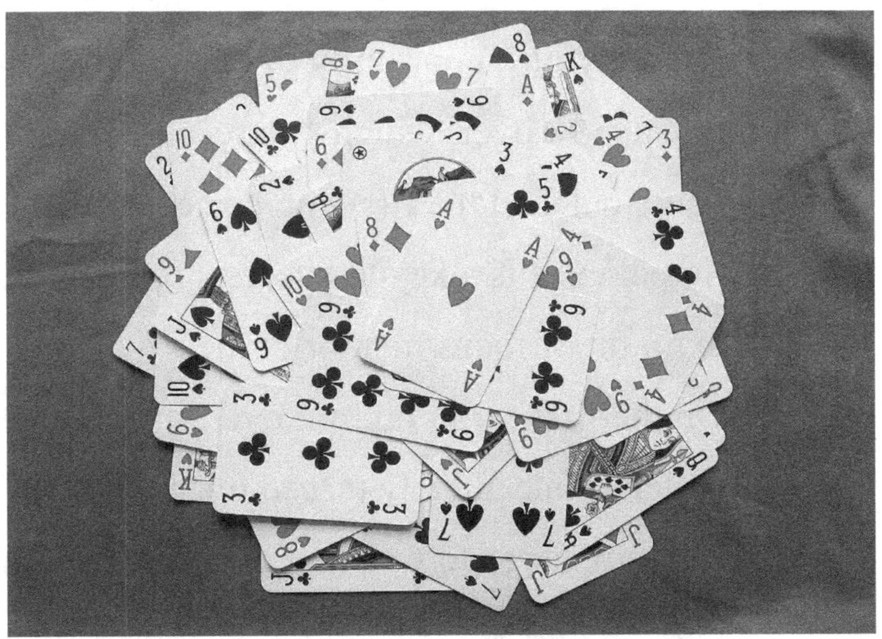

32a

<u>There are very many of this type of card game on the market.</u>

But, let's say you only have a couple of decks of ordinary playing cards!

Off into the Garden you all go and sit in a circle with the cards inside you, within reasonable reach of everybody – if not get the kids to do some of the reaching for the elderly!

    a) Singly, in Pairs, or even Groups!
    b) Match the Number and Suit exactly;
    c) Or, Just match the Colour;
    d) Or Just match the Number.
    e) For those not familiar with any rules, here are ours:

i. <u>First, lay all the cards you are playing with, scattered about, **face down**</u>.

ii. On your go you turn only 2 cards over, *one at a time*.

iii. If you make a pair you continue with another 2...

iv. *Not two at once*, as that will mean you will have missed your opportunity of matching with a previous one turned over, which you recall, all too late, would have matched the first you turned over.

v. So patience is a key to success; it also gives you that extra bit of focus/memory time.

vi. On the first card you turn over, try to remember if it matches one already turned over.

vii. If you manage to turn that one over and make a pair, they go into your accumulative pile.

viii. You then have another turn and continue until you fail to make a pair the beauty of the game is the variable pairing rules above.

ix. Also, you can go mega, and play with more than one pack laid face down before you!

x. The person/team with the most cards retrieved, wins!

OFF YOU GO TRY ME

<u>PEANUT BUTTER/JAM JAR PICKLES:</u>

These two final games (which can be played indoors & out) were prompted by >>>

i the image of greed which doesn't always pay;

ii the thought of a certain experiment with monkies

iii And, lastly what President Trump epitomises!

1st.   **<u>Greed:-</u>** So, for me it conjures up a picture of Pooh Bear

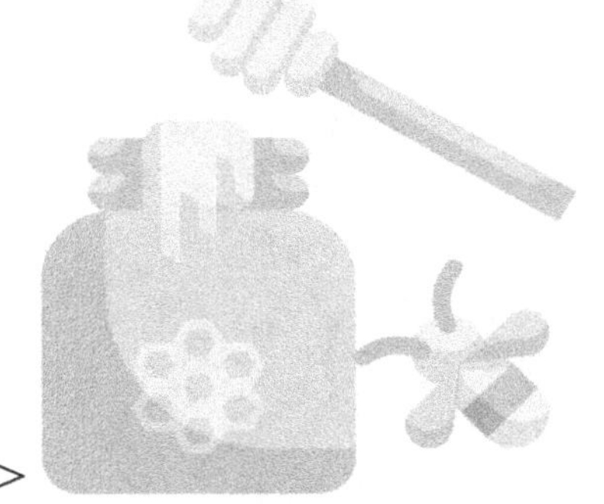

with his hand in the Honey jar >>

34

2nd.   **<u>Monkey Experiment:-</u>** Continuing the Honet Pot greed

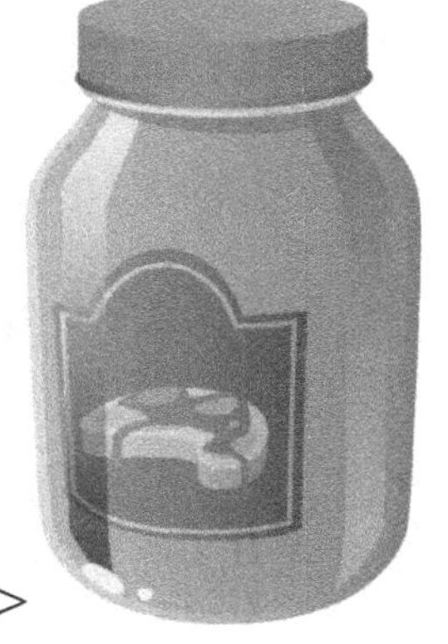

image I considered this as a neat example >>

35

3rd.   The third symbolises what Donald stands for: that
Commercial Success is his & America's driving force to the Top
of The World Pile! But, one ingredient/asset for any good
businessman is his bartering ability and this will figure in one of
the following games to show the younger element it's not what
you haven't got and want that is important to others, it is what
they want and haven't got, but you have!

AND SO TO THE GAMES>>>> You can make these more difficult,
though perhaps more annoying for some who might give up, that is
the usage of plastic milk bottles (+ cap) and marbles?

Up to you!

So, off we go, jar in hand!

11:- *24, Balloons & 33 + 34 jars above (plastic preferred).*

    a. There is one qualification for the jar: its neck must be
narrower that the jar below, as the pictures depict and the
cap has an important part to play also.

    b. When Monkies tried this their greed got the better of them
and they couldn't understand, at first, why their hand went
in so easily, but wouldn't come out when there was/were a
sweet/sweets in their grasp?

    c. Here too, is that lesson which the younger element must
learn.

    d. It can be played in teams and to add difficulty the amount
of sweets increases after each round!

e. The Honey/Peanut butter jar sizes are for the kids, but as stated above,the more difficult aspect is where you play with marbles and the much narrower necked plastic milk bottles – where marbles = sweets in the final outcome.

f. At the 'outcome' end stage the art of *'bartering'* might come into its own!?

g. So off we go >> Let's assume the jar holds 30 max...

   i. We start with a plastic bowl, preferably just smaller than enough to suffiicently hold all 30 assorted sweets comfortably, without effort on the player's part! Work up the age range so the youngster starts with say 15.

   ii. Put 15 in the bowl; place the not too tightly at all, closed jar upside down, in front of the child, with instructions to start on the word go (When the stop watch also starts – found on so many I-Phones nowadays have this facility)!

   iii. The child must open the jar and put all the sweets inside; close the jar lid and stand it upside down in the place it started.

   iv. The next in line then reverses the process and without picking the jar up too far so he/she cannot start pouring them out into the bowl, must, again with no pouring out, get the sweets out of the jar back into the bowl, without any falling from it, which has since has 5 added – making 20.

v. The jar then must be replaced and the jar returned to its inverted state.

vi. The next empties etc as 5 more are addd etc. until 30 in the bowl is reached– simple so far, but not over and here comes the maths educational part, if there is a number of youngsters playing (? Against the elders?) where no help is given by the elders:

vii. The next must only take out 25 and put back into the jar etc , then the next takes out/ puts back in the bowl 20 and so the final one takes out 15 and puts them back in the jar; places the jar in its inverted state and the timer is then stopped!

viii. If there are any bright sparks out there you will have realised the secret short cut: rather than counting out until 15, 20, or whatever, just leave five by your side and you should be certain that what is left is the number you need return! HUSH!

ix. **I'm sure you can adapt & embellish upon the above.**

x. The Sweets? Bartering? No, I haven't forgotten.

xi. Whether played individually, or in teams this process is the same and just as much *'tormenting'* fun!

xii.   Say the winning team of three from the 30 gets **6** sweets each; the losers **4** sweets each; the sweet allocation is not simply to hand out **6** each and **4** each accordingly – Oh No! Because people have their favourites and this was a family favourite candy/sweet <u>assortment</u> say like Cadbury's???

xiii.   So the youngest in the winning team takes his/her first choice; the next youngest his/hers etc; then we go to the losing team who picks their first choice in age order. Then we go onto the 2nd choices etc...

xiv.   Now if one of the losing team knows that somebody in the winning team favours sweet X, and there is another one or two available, he/she picks this with the thought that if so popular the person wanting it most would give more than one sweet in exchange? We'd make a trump ourt of them yet – if the parent so wishes? **But sweets are such a draw!**

OFF YOU GO TRY ME

LETTING OFF STEAM GETTING WET:

FROM ABOVE ↑ >>>

> *Anyhow, I have a less dangerous wet usage for the balloons!*

AND HERE IT IS ↓ >>> **FIRST THE BIG BOYS**

From A1b above:- Again for those who need let off some juvenile steam... *01, Paddling Pool 07, Tennis Balls etc.10, Footballs Hard 14, Shuttlecocks15, Ping Pong Balls 24 Balloons.*

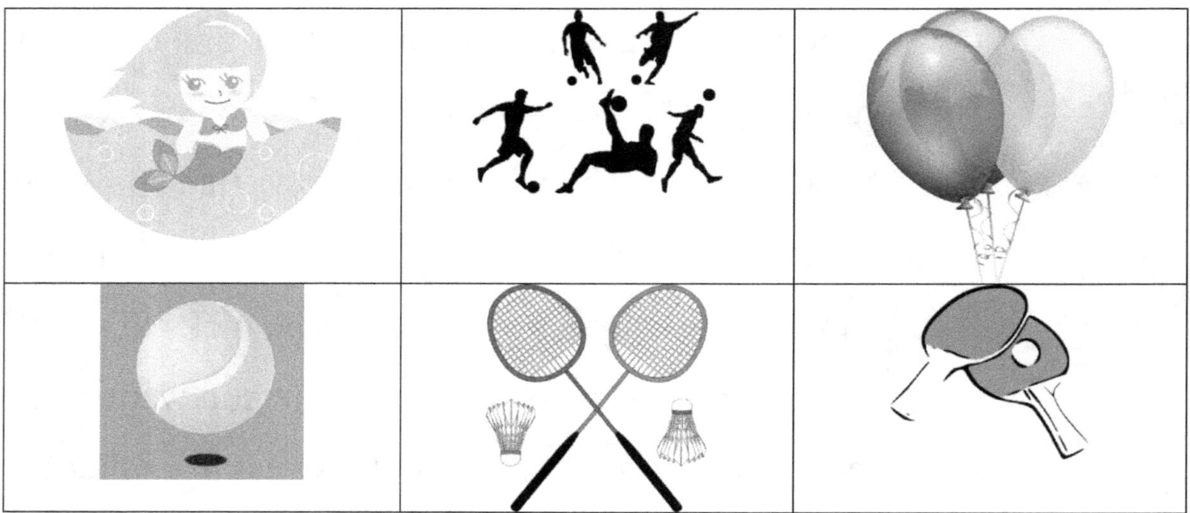

a. Keep the paddling pool

b. Put into it all the ping pong balls you have

c. Also all the shuttlecocks you have which will float there

d. Fill up your remaining balloons with water

e. Can be a Team v Team, but more likely those who think much of themselves as good shots standing off against their main opponent

f. Those not playing can still sweet bet on who will score first/last/most...

g. Scoring is simply the knocking out of the pool any of the objects floating within

h. So each standing opposite each other, within a prescribed square area behind the pool (4<>6m^2 suggested to keep them on their toes when bombarded by balloons/balls!).

i. The player(s) awaits the other's balloon volley, which he/she will return, hoping to score knocking something out!

j. When the balloons are exhausted/burst then it is onto the tennis balls

k. Finally throwing the football(s)

l. Should you have poor throwers ensure you have a time limit imposed.

m. Invariably it is likely the contestants will get wet

n. The spectators unlikely so long as prudently they place themselves well to the sides!

FROM ABOVE ↑ >>>

<u>Anyhow, I have a less dangerous wet usage for the balloons!</u>

AND HERE IT IS ↓ >>> **<u>SECOND THE LITTLE BOYS+GIRLS</u>**

A Kiddie's Brave/frightening Alternative Addition:

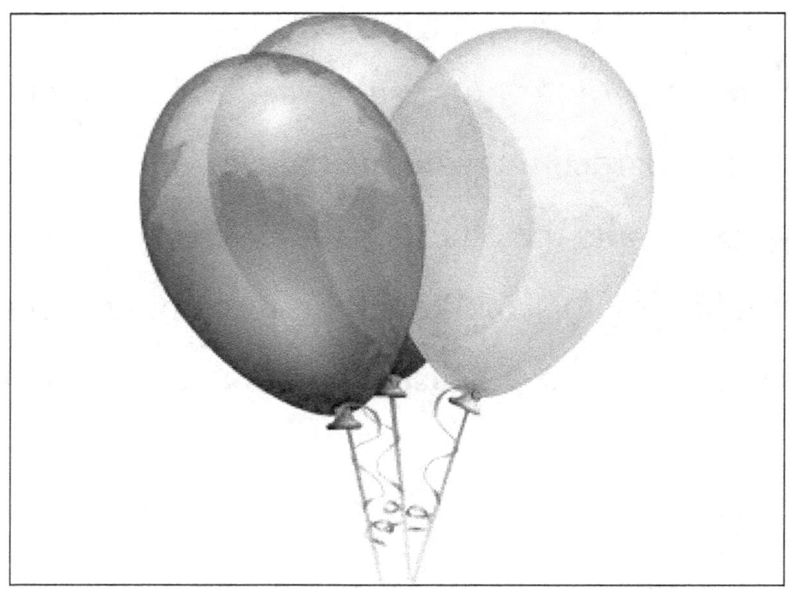

If you don't need to use the filled balloons this way, you can create the excitement & a little trepidation for the younger ones by ... you guessed it...

Catching the balloons for sweet prizes (If they dare?)

For there is always the fear of being splashed all over!

So, it's best to do this on a nice warm day.

Happy Drenching!

OFF YOU GO TRY ME

<u>**And here I must give special thanks & mention to all those who supplied the 'artistic' pictorial support through the book and perhaps in my small way I can put business their way:-**</u>

Pages	Item	Contributor
~31+	Sporty Caption	Thanks to Pixaby OpenClipart-Vectors (**All Sports**) pictograms-159824_1280
~34+	1= Paddling Pool Mermaid	Thanks to pixabay Gogry **paddling pool** mermaid-4299707_1280
~34+	2= Watering Can	Thanks to pixabay Clipart-Vectors **watering-can-**146445_1280
~34+	3= Washing Clothes Line	Thanks Clicker-Free-Vector-Images-**clothesline-**308496_1280
~34+	4= Red Bucket Cleaning Wash	Thanks Pixabay Prographer_ **bucket-1643406_1280**
~35+	5a=Plastic Containers	Thanks to Pixabay 200degrees **soap-2181046_1280 Plastic**
~35+	5b= Plastic Bottles	Thanks to pixabay Clker-free-vector-images **(plastic) drinks bottles**-33601_1280
~35+	6= Wheelchair Ramp System	Thanks Clker-Free-Vector-Images **ramp** for wheelchair-43877_1280
~36+	7= Balls Tennis	Thanks to pixabay AlLes **balls tennis**-1477297_1280
~36+	8= Golf Club	Thanks Clker-Free-Vector-Images **club and ball golf-**32262_1280
~36+	9= Golf Balls	Thanks Pixabay 47ronin47 **Wedge club golf-**284633_1280
~37+	10= Footballs	Thanks Clipart Mohamed-hassan **football-**2755481_1280
~37+	11= Tennis Racquets	Thanks Clipart-Vectors **tennis (racquet)** -309617_1280
~38+	12= Badminton Racquets	Thanks Pixabay BilliTheCat **Badminton (racquets)** graphic-4067696_1280
~38+	13= Net for Badminton	Thanks to pixabay Clker-Free-Vector-Images **badminton net** or volleyball-33404_1280
~38+	14= Badminton Shuttlecocks	Thanks Open Clipart-Vectors **shuttlecock** badminton-159415_1280
~39+	15= Table Tennis Bats & Balls	Thanks to Pixabay Clker-free-vector-images **table tennis balls +bat**s-25764_1280
~39+	16= Ball of String	Thanks to pixabay B0red **string ball**-2136167_1280
~39+	17= Cricket Stumps	Thanks Clipart-Vectors **cricket**-155965_1280 **(Stumps)**
~40+	17b=Cricket Bat	Thanks Open Clipart-Vectors **cricket- (bat)** 150560_1280

~40+	18= Darts Board	*Thanks Pixabay Zeppi2002* **dart-board**-*4679593_1280*
~40+	18a= Darts Play (With a Warning!)	*Thanks Pixabay Pixel2013* **darts injury** *person - 3076079_1920 (slightly ~~cut~~ cropped) Ouch!*
~41+	19= Darts	*Thanks Pixabay BilliTheCat* **darts** *graphic-3997742_1280*
~41+	20= Water Pistol	*Thanks Pixabay iamyesarun* **water pistol** *water-4144817_1280*
~41+	21= Marbles	*Thanks Clipart Couleur* **marbles**-*1659398_1920*
~42+	22= Wheelie Bins	*Thanks to Hans Braxmeier Pixabay* **dustbin-(Wheelie Bins)** *95178_1920*
~42+	22a = That Gap	**Self's Wheelie Bins Adj** *showing That Gap*
~42+	23= Wheelie Bin Liners	*Thanks Pixabay Councelling* **liner** *for garbage-can-535156_1920*
~43+	24= Balloons	*Thanks Clker-Free-Vector-Images* **balloons**-*25737_1280*
~43+	25= Cardboard Boxes (Amazon!?)	*Thanks to Pixabay Mediamodifier* **boxes** *businessman-2108029_1920*
~43+	26= Knitting Needles + Yarn	*Thanks to pixabay Clker-Free-Vector-Images* **knitting needles yarn**-*309401_1280*
~44+	27= Used Drink Cans (In Tact!)	*Thanks to Pixabay Clker-free- vector-images* **cans** *six-pack-25200_1280*
~44+	28= Hockey Sticks as Bat Substitutes	*Thanks to Pixabay KeithJJ field-* **hockey-(stick)** *1537396_1920*
~44+	29= Used Paint Pots	*Thanks to Clipart-Vectors* **paint pots** *color-161088_1280*
~45+	30= We can: All Age Involvement	*Thanks OpenClipart-Vectors adults golf-146964_1280*
~45+	31= Scissors Tape etc.	*Thanks to Pexels Jess Bailey* **tape** **_etc_** *blue-***scissors**-*1117542*
~45+	32= Our Up-Side Down Game Fun	*Thanks to creative commons stockvault-***upside-down***195816*
~97+	32a= Pack(s) of Cards Choice Fun	*Thanks to Wikimedia Commons*
~60+	33= Lacrosse Stick Adaptation	*Thanks to Wikimedia Commons*
~99+	34= Honey Pot	*Thanks to Pixabay DoomSlayer's Honey Pot & bee-5069122_1280*
~99+	35= Peanut Butter Jar	*Thanks Pixabay OpenClipart-Vectors peanut-butter-576887_1280*

AND

NOW FOR THE BIGGER CHALLENGING EVENTS WHERE THE PARENTS/GRANDPARENTS WILL HAVE THEIR ORGANISING INGENUITY CAPABILITY TESTED TO THE FULL

BUT
NOT AS MUCH AS THE GREAT WHO-DUNNIT ESCAPADE IN MY,

WHO STOLE OUR CHRISTMAS PRESENTS?
SCREAMED SETH & JUDE!
V3 – THE THREE DAY <u>HEISTS</u>

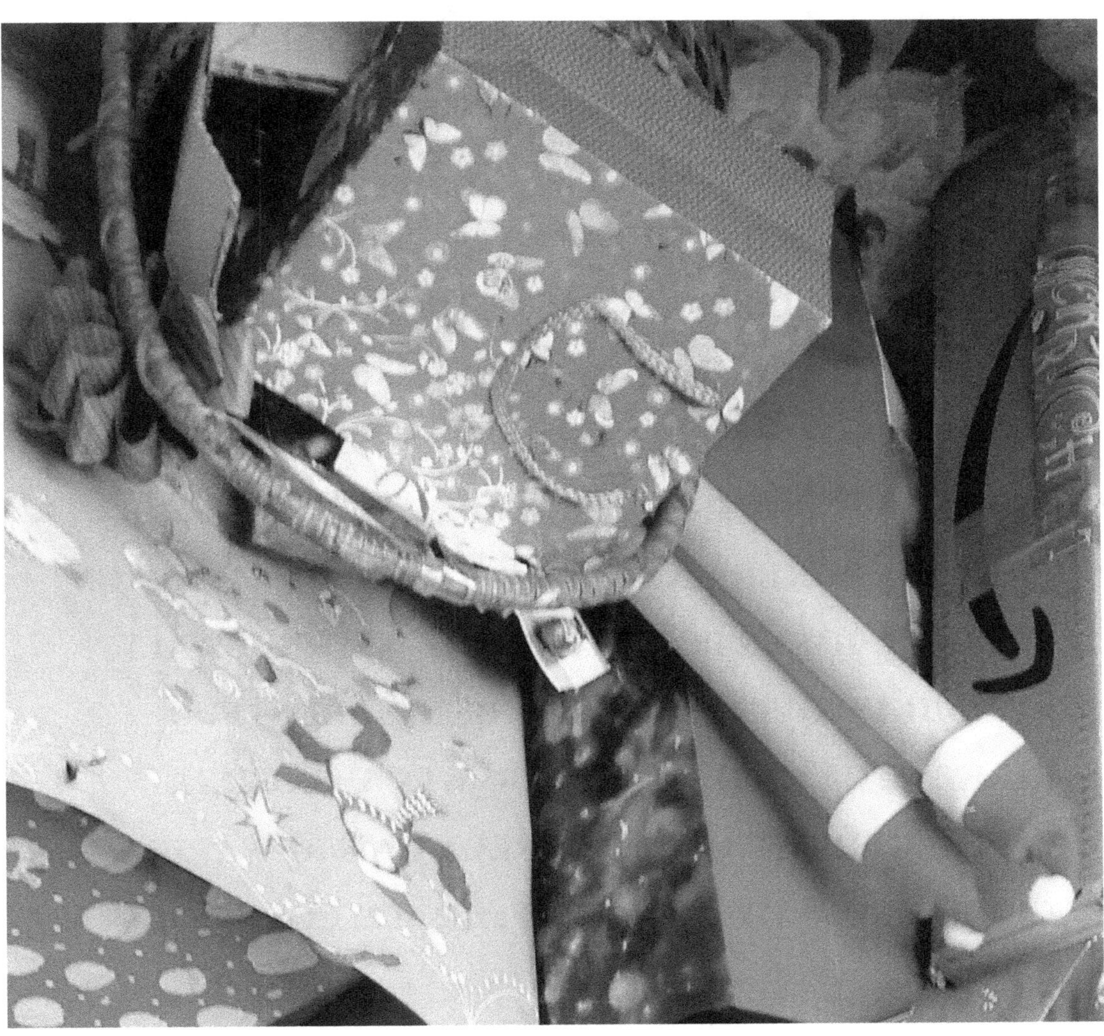

<u>**NB**</u>**:** *Any item below tagged as (I = indoor) & (O = outdoor activity)*
(I/O = Both) (B = Birthdays) (HSG = Home/Social gatherings)(X = Xmas)

1st.   **YULETIDE > PM EASY DOES IT FOR THE GUEST(S)**   *X*

2nd.   **BIRTHDAY:- THAT (POST PARTY) CAKE DETOUR!** *I/O*

3rd.   **CHRISTMAS > PRIZE DAY PRESENT GUESSING TIME!?**   *I*

4th.   **BIRTHDAY > FREE (CHOCOLATE/SWEET) FOR A ?** *O*

5th.   **BIRTHDAY > BRING ME A BALL FOR A SWEET GAME** *O*

6th.   **A JACK & THE GIANT CHALLENGING ESCAPADE!**   *O*

7th.   **CHRISTMAS MYA'S CAKE (Part 1 of 2) BAKING**   *I*

8th.   **CAKE BAKING SIMPLE MYA MINGLING MAKING**   *I*

9th.   **SOCIAL GATHERING YOUNG & OLD PRIZE MIXES!**   *I*

   10th.   **FOR LADIES EYES ONLY**

11th. **A GROUP HELLO - WHO ARE YOU AGAIN?**   *I/O*

12th. **A GROUP HELLO - WHAT ARE YOU AGAIN?**   *I/O*

13th. **XMAS CAKE MAKING INNER SECRETS REVEALED**   *I*

14th. **GARDENING CAN BE FUN BUT THE SPELLING NEVER**   *I/O*

15th. **BRIDGE A GAP A TRAVEL GAMBLE INTERLUDE**   *I*

16th. **BRIDGE A POKER HAND MAKE THE MOST OF A PACK**   *I*

17th. **BRIDGE A JOKER POKER PACK RE-ASSEMBLE ALL**   *I*

18th. **RUMMIKUB/QUIDDLER – MATHS/SPELLING FUN**   *I/O*

19th. **KIRKE – THE CARD GAME YOU WIN BY LOSING!**   *I*

20th. **CAR REGISTRATION Nos SO RELAXING/REWARDING** *O*

21st. **CHRISTMAS > MYA'S CAKE (Part 2 of 2) COVERING**   *X/I*

Well, I touched upon Easter & Birthdays before, But, and it is that Ultimate No Doubt But, Christmas is the Biggie for ALL kids and so this occasion has Pride & Place with the **attention** (to detail) it truly deserves!

This memorable time that is Christmas:

The later productions work well

if you have more than one child

And at least one of the children

Has reached a *reasonable reading stage*.

<u>**1 YULETIDE**</u>**:- (PM EASY DOES IT) FOR THE GUEST(S)!**

Kids were not the only ones who should get the special treatment: some (certain deserving) adults who (less fortunate) couldn't afford to bring large/expensive presents would therefore be embarrassed to receive them, or those who just felt embarrassed if made a fuss over. I've always felt they merited, special (undercover, or should that be underhand) treatment.
After lunch a lucky number allocated to each person for future reference/raffle use.

A Rigged Raffle!
The raffle reference, above, is another sneaky way you can ensure your deserving case gets the star treatment.

Simplicity, this, and no sleight of hand needed!

By arranging a free raffle with a bumper prize going to this pre-arranged winner – (the number, between 1 & ?? = the number of attendees) the number that is allocated to the deserving case is the winner! Hoorah – success achieved!
How?
All (say) 12 folded tickets which had been placed in a bag/ hat to be drawn were the same as the number you gave to you-know-who, earlier that day!
These must all be destroyed as soon as the winning ticket is produced.

She/he is so astoundedly grateful, (even more so if he/she won at bingo)!
My scam went unnoticed until one of my twins asked me in later life – all then had to be revealed, not before I had replicated the *ploy* a couple of times thereafter.
OFF YOU GO TRY ME

2 <u>BIRTHDAY</u>:- THAT (POST PARTY) CAKE DETOUR!

But, kids were my great love and at the twins' (then grand-children's) parties I would be the one to distribute the goodie-bags at the end of the occasion: ever/still the fun creator and quiz master.

<u>Goodie Bag Finalé</u>: If one or two individuals arrived, before the main bunch, I would say they had to try to pick the bag (of the only three/four supposedly) which contained a large piece of birthday cake.

– I revelled in the sight of those glad faces, who, seemingly, made the right choice against all the odds!

AS did all the subsequent pickers!

Simplicity >< <u>I ensured all bags contained a large piece of cake</u>!

OFF YOU GO TRY ME

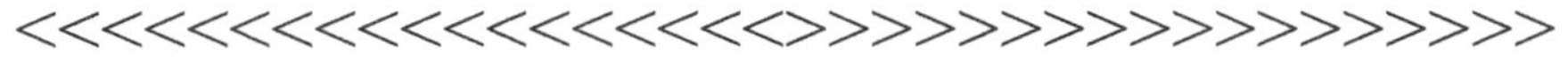

NOW FOLLOWS

The First of the

Mammoth

'SPECIAL DAY'

Productions!

<u>Not for the faint-hearted</u>

(Grand)/Parent(s)!

Nor those,

who are not into fine detail

And ***sneaky tactics***!

Good Directing is Key(1)
Any Spielberg in your Family?

+

Good Mis-Directing is Key(2)
Any Magicians in your Family?

Confused again?

<u>Well, here goes nothing...</u>

OFF YOU GO TRY ME **IF YOU DARE!!!**

>>>

3 <u>CHRISTMAS</u> PRIZE DAY PRESENT GUESSING TIME!?

(Labels/Envelopes prep time 20 minutes) + (Extra selection of Prize Presents (See 9)

If you are one of those families who do not celebrate Christmas Day/Dinner together, followed by presents' distribution, then this might not be for you: it will all become apparent as I explain.

This you'll find is another novel way the kids can celebrate/share those present giving moments AND all ages can participate in the fun.

1. *Don't Circulate that **<u>this year none of the presents you, the family host/hostess, are giving away will have a name label on them</u>** —they will be become a post-dinner gift-guessing game time!*

2. *Leave the surprise to when all other presents/parcels have been handed out.*

3. *Those children who can read can take it in turns to be the Distributor Judges ^{DJ} unless it is their turn to guess.*

4. *The unlabelled family gifts kept separate from the rest (say in an upstairs bedroom) will be the last to be distributed. NB make sure they are not in the room allocated for coats etc to be left in, otherwise the surprise will be spoiled!*

5. *These special parcel items will have a sealed plain brown envelope ↓ stuck to each with the name of the recipient inside.*

6. *A pile of the labels, which would normally be attached to the gift parcels, is then laid before the guests – obviously the host &/or hostess gifts are not part of this game.*

7. *Decide who is to guess first (The Chooser) – or pick a card (Ace High)!*

8. *One of the [DJ] Children then goes out with the Host/Hostess. He/she then views the presents; selects one (+ See PS below) and brings it down for the next Chooser waiting to decide whose it is.*

   a. *He/She then passes His/Her chosen Label over to the Child [DJ], whilst the Host opens the envelope attached to the present.*

   b. *The Host + Child then check to see if the label is an exact match – so if the present is for two people jointly, then only picking a label with only one name on it will not count! This is because some are joint presents – just to confuse even more – say Mum & Dad, or Son & Dad etc....*

9. *If the Chooser is correct, He/She can pick one of the Prizes the Host/Hostess has laid out extra for any such winners: Something akin to a Christmas Hamper Contents e.g. Spirit Miniatures (for Adults), or Chocolates/Sweets (for the Children), select food stuffs – even small batched £1 or £2 coins (for Kids who want to save up for something in the future of their choice!)*

10. *This selection ratio of extra prizes to gifts, to make it tempting, especially at the end [B] should be around 2 >1!*

11. *The Present recipient is handed their Package.*

12. *If the Chooser is correct, He/She then also retains the right to make another Present Label Match Choice.*

13.   *If the Chooser is incorrect then it is the turn of the next in line Chooser.*

14.   *Continue until all the presents have been given out.*

15.   *It will be that your extra prize gifts will not get all used up, and so when you are down to your last Label Match Choice, here ^B if the Chooser is correct, He/She wins all that is left: failing this it will be the last Present Recipient who wins all! Sometimes here ^B the Booty can be substantial!*

16.   *The beauty in this is again the happy kid helter-skelter up/down the stairs; the responsibility given to him/her to make the next present choice; their excited involvement when it is their turn to be a Chooser; the life education that they cannot always be a Winner!*

17.   *Although, if unlucky, then I'm sure the ultimate winner(s) will ensure they get something they like from the Hamper (See also variation below ^{XXX})*

18.   *Fun Warning: As the idea of all this is to confuse, I have found Old Biscuit Tins, padded inside, a great way of hiding the identity of any medium sized present within – so having a feel will get the Chooser no closer to the answer!*

19.   *Alternatively, put a smaller present rolled up in several layers of newspaper inside a much larger cardboard box – this will be the kids' first port of call, thinking the biggest is always for them!*

But it won't be, will it!

Have Fun!

<u>I always do!</u>

PS The astute amongst you will have suggested that if you keep score of who has received a present, then you can likely guess who's left?!

But my/your *get-around-this* is that you always ensure there is more than one present for certain individuals, and at least two of these 'extras' should always be the last ones to be brought in by the *DJ Child!*

Sly Eh?

BOUNCY CASTLES ARE SO EXPENSIVE TO HIRE!

AND SO HERE WE ARE ON SOME YOUNG CHILD'S

BIRTHDAY – BOUNCY CASTLE=LESS

THANKFULLY IT IS A HOT SUNNY DAY

AND NOW IT IS THAT BIG REVEAL

DISTRACTION TIME

AS ALL THE YOUNG ATTENDEES

ARE TOLD TO SIT DOWN

AND AWAIT THEIR

'*<u>BIRTHDAY TUMMY TO BE FED</u>*
<u>*WET ADVENTURE TIME!*</u>'

STORY TIME WITH A DIFFERENCE!?

<u>JACK AND THE BEANSTALK</u>

<u>BUT ITS MYA BIG BUT:-</u>

<u>WITH 'STOMACH PRECIOUS'</u>

<u>CHOCOLATES AND/or SWEETS + ICE CREAMS!</u>

>>>>>>>>>>

BUT FIRST A

4 <u>BIRTHDAY</u> A FREE (CHOCOLATE/SWEET)
FOR A BALL) FORTUNE FOR ALL!

1. *Get all the kids to go to end of the garden;*

2. *and turn their back to you – then*

3. *Tell them to close their eyes.*

4. **'To get a free chocolate/sweet you must...**

5. **Bring any 2 balls to me**

6. **So take your pick.**

7. **When I tell you NOW**

8. **Then you look for 2 balls to bring me.**

9. *Here you should bring a few more balls than kids!*

10. *(I fortunately belong to a Tennis Club and the used ones are sold cheaply to whoever wants them!) #*

11. *Similarly a few more chocolates/sweets!*

12. *The best I find are Milky Way Stars. #*

13. *There again there are Mini Bite Size Animals? #*

14. *And my numerical mainstay Dolly Mixtures! #*

15. *Scatter balls about the lawn and walkways*

16. *And so many behind things!*

17. *Not your flower areas!*

18. *Especially no balls adjacent any prickly plants!*

19.   Then after their first chocolate

20.   TheY will be eager for more....

<u>(The small size chocolate/sweets are especially chosen to avoid sugar overload!?)</u> #↑

<u>But as with all kids functions always precheck for any allergies – here lactose intolerant!</u>

<u>AND you could use the small chocolates + sweets left overs to add to the Goody Bags!</u> # # *(see end)*

If you have a marker pen then you can adapt/add to the

>>>>>>>>>>>>>>>>>>>

5 BIRTHDAY > BRING ME A BALL FOR A SWEET GAME:-

1. *As each child brings you their 2 balls – mark their shortened name on the outside – this will be the ball they ultimately take home, BUT, these balls can be part of the follow up game!*
2. *Make sure each child knows their balls from the rest, then,*
3. *Tell them all again to turn their backs to you and count to 20 slowly...*
4. *As you hide the balls in series...*
5. *This means if there are say six playing then you will have 12 balls*
6. *These you hide in clusters of 3 near to each other.*
7. *So there are only four hiding places to avoid some individual balls being hidden is some more awkward than others places!*
8. *And so yet again 2 balls = 2 sweets!*
9. *So once again to reiterate the smaller the sweets the better!*

AND SO ONTO YOUR EVER LARGER CHALLENGING ESCAPADE BUT BOTH CAN BE FOR LARGE GATHERINGS

6 BIRTHDAY > *A JACK & THE GIANT ESCAPADE!*

1. *Get the kids together seated in a huddle.*

2. ***Then ask if any of them know the 'Jack & The Beanstalk Story?***

3. *Await responses then briefly add your own interpretation as follows:-*

4. ***Well my story is similar there is a boy who tries to steal a Giant's Gold Treasure & his Gold Laying Chicken***

5. ***BUT***

6. ***I have no chicken which lays gold!***

7. ***I also have no gold, but I have found something you'll want.***

8. ***The story boy is called Jack, but today we will call him/her ???***

9. *(Here you use the name of the birthday boy/girl) – Say today it's*

10. **Little Jude and the Giant,** *(for our story unfolding – below)..*

11. *Now the equipment....*

12. *And here you need improvise if you do not have either of these..*

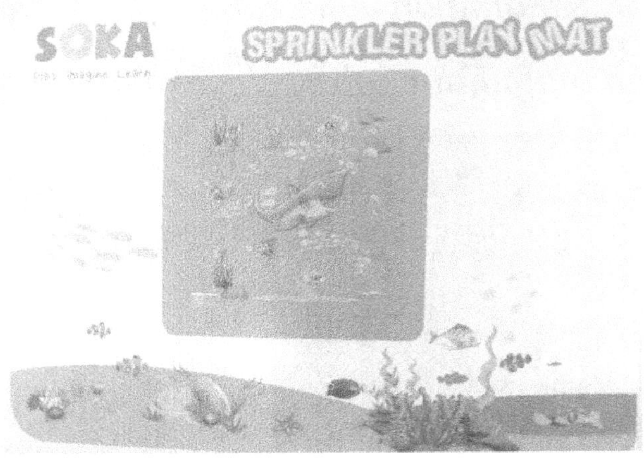

13.

14.   *EG a SOKA = <u>Large Square Sprinkle and Splash Water Play Mat Sprinkler Splash Pad Summer Spray Inflatable Water Toy for Kids Dogs Pets and Outdoor Garden Family Activities</u>*

OR

15.   *Failing such a contraption, a simple Rotating Garden Sprinkler.*

16.   *Then something which resembles <u>a castle top with steps in and a slide out</u>, or <u>an offground playhouse/playset</u> with steps in and a slide out, or playset with steps in and a slide out.*

17.   *Like this one*

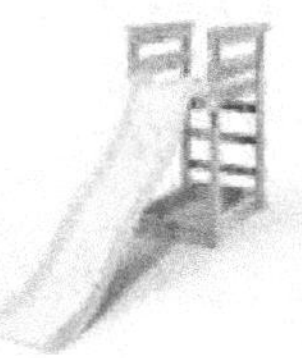

18.   *by REBO*

19.   *If none of these, something not too dangerous to climb over*

20.   ***AND***

21.   *<u>Any of these but with some area below/beside</u> where kids can sit and be contained.*

22.   *Depending on your garden size and contents, if you also have an outbuilding obstacle around which the kids have to run around...*

23.   *And to slow them down some thing like a longish crawl tunnel*

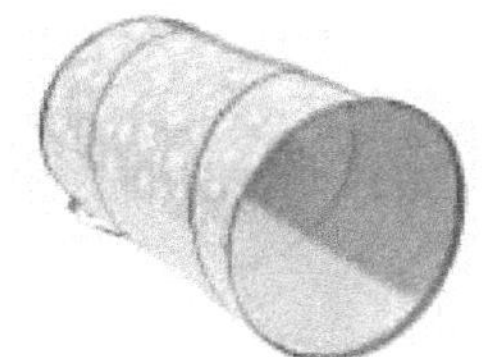

24. *This by Chad Valley*

25. *The best is one with a peeka-boo hole on the top-(see why later)*

26. *So Stage Set off we go...back to Little John's Story...*

27. **In Jack & The Beanstalk there was giant who didn't want anyone going after his gold** *– pause –*

28. **BUT**

29. **You all are the children he has captured trying...**

30. **But he is kind as he doesn't want you to go without food.**

31. **And so he feeds you 3 times a day >>**

32. **Breakfast, Lunch and Dinner.**

33. **So, who here likes more chocolate?**

34. *Await responses...*

35. **Raise your hands Who wants a chocolate**

36. *Await responses...Then again*

37. **Answer me yes or no...**

38. *After their yes*

39. **All those who want a chocolate shout out yes please!**

40. *Await responses...Then*

41. **All those who want 2 chocolates shout out yes please!**

42. *After their yes*

43. **All those who want 3 chocolates shout out yes please!**

44. **BUT**

45. *TELL THEM*

46. ***Sorry, there is one thing stopping me and it is <u>the Giant!</u>***

47. <u>*Then allocate this role to Little Jude's Dad/Grandad?*</u>

48. <u>*Even give him a monster's mask!?*</u>

49. ***And you are all his prisoners!***

50. ***Making sure you are then all in his penned area.***

51. ***But you are lucky Little Jude has agreed he feeds you all.***

52. ***Do you remember I offered you each 3 chocolates?***

53. ***These will be your three meals for today.***

54. ***BUT***

55. ***Your cruel Giant Dad/Granded will not make it easy for you!***

56. ***I have chocolates for you all but***

57. ***Imagine <u>he has hidden me some where else in his castle</u>***

58. *Then walk away behind them, or some place so not to obstruct*

59. ***He has set a trap out for you and obstacles to get around.***

60. *Here you need to have pre-thought out a long way around –*

61. *About the garden, about any large outbuilding – improvise where you can but nothing where they can trip and fall.*

62. *Get your local Giant to run the course omitting the Soka above*

63. ***BUT***

64. *And here comes the First Big But they must first overcome*

65. *That Soka/sprinkler system meaning they all will get a little wet*

66. *Ensure they cannot get around it and must jump through/over it.*

67. *Blow it up using your garden hose attachment and ensure it works with a large wide or tall spray.*

68. *Now tell the kids **'I have 3 chocolates for each of you'***

69. *(I use Milky Way Stars #↑ or something that size)*

70. **But the Giant has proclaimed you can only have one at a time at each meal**

71. **And you must go around the way he just showed you**

72. **BUT**

73. **You must also go/jump through his water trap**

74. *Bring it out already water filled then connect up to the supply*

75. **If you don't then Boo Hoo no FOOD for you!**

76. **So hold up your hands if you want to try to get your food!**

77. *Await response – hopefully there are no spoil sports?*

78. **Then after the water trap go around the rest of the garden**

79. *Here ensure an adult or two makes sure they stick to the course*

80. **Now to be fair I have a bag with your names inside except**

81. **You can only go when I call your name...**

82. *Little Birthday Boy Jude (who you know loves this sort of thing) goes first – call his name automatically*

83. **Now who's to follow him ???** *pulling a name from the bag*

84. *And to encourage him/her get the group to chant his/her name*

85. *"Go Jenny/Jude/Jeremy or whoever!"*

86. *As they come to the end you will give them a chocolate*

87. *then off they will go again...*

88. *"Go Jenny/Jude/Jeremy or whoever!"*

89. **BUT**

90. **The second and third times you must go through his castle and hope he doesn't try to stop you.**

91. *This means (if you have something with steps up and a slide down) they have to go up and down this before they reach the water. (An example is as shown in No 18 above)*

92. *Here your giant can wait at the bottom of the slide*

93. *With legs wide apart which the children will slide between*

94. *AND he can make a vain effort to catch them as they pass by*

95. *When the last one passes through for the third time switch off the sprinkler.*

96. *At the end then ask if they enjoyed it and let them calm down within/beneath the Playset/Castle building.*

97. *Perhaps towel down any who want it.*

98. *If your kids structure is on two floors, (As No 18 above) put the boys beneath the girls if possible, but for safety reasons don't put too many on top.*

99. *My other reason here is that my climbing frame with steps up and a slide down, has an area which with cross battens can double up as a prison which needs clambering out of, which boys excel at, and no doubt in this equality era so many girls do too!*

100. *Leave them there to compose themselves for the next challenge!*

101. ***Now dear children image your giant has had his dinner***

102. ***<u>This is your chance to escape with some of his Treasure Chest full of his prize ice cream</u>***

103. *Here you need get enough of the same ice cream which all will enjoy – for any lactose * intolerant then make the necessary arrangement...*

104. *I use Magnums Ice Cream Sticks – you can buy the standard or mini sizes whatever...but suggest the smaller to avoid sugar overload!?*

105. ***There is a Bar for each of you – they are all the same (*except)***

106. ***So only take one***

107. ***BUT***

108. *Take the Soka Mat and reposition it more centrally in the garden*

109. *Place the magnums on it right in the middle!*

110. *Here you need reset your Soka/Sprinkler system*

111. *Switch on to maximum!*

112. ***BUT***

113. ***To escape and take a magnum for yourself you will have to get wet again***

114. ***BUT***

115. ***To escape you need go down the slide then through the tube tunnels and out the other end through the sleepy giant's legs***

116. *This is why I like the tunnel to have an opening on top so the Giant hover above it & can make some futile effort to catch the young prisoner escapee by trying to grab him, or her, through this opening. (Tech Traders have one on Amazon) (As do Chad Valley)...*

117. *If there is none with an upper opening the Giant should position himself at the end facing down where the child is escaping, again making a futile NOISY grab...*

118. *If you have 2 crawl tubes then he can position himself over either*

119. *Or even both if running after the child!*

120. *Or he can have a servant helper at the other tube he's not at* *

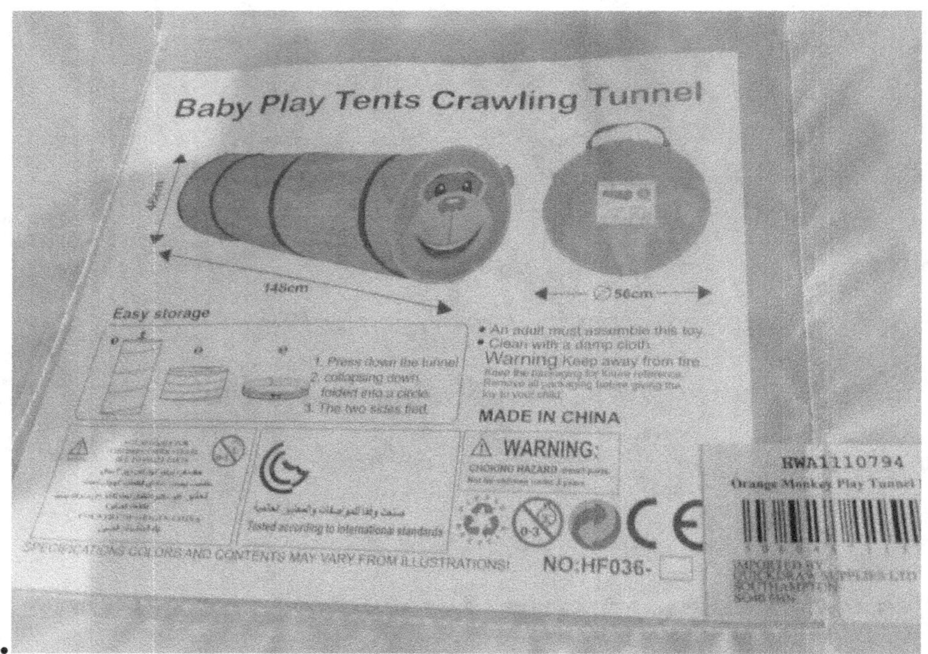

121.

122. *Additionally to show the Giant is prevented from running after the children have each of his legs tied to the handles of ..*

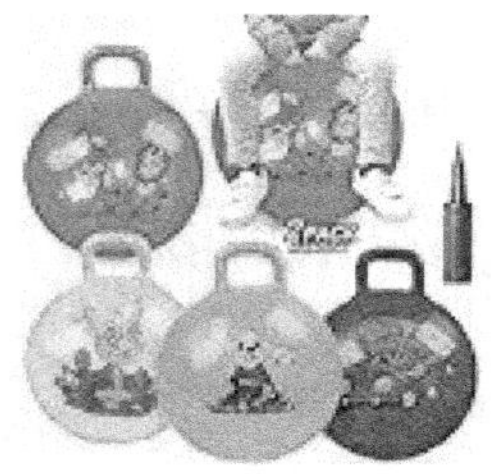

Hymaz 2 Pack Choice of Bouncy Hopper, with 18 inch handles...

123. *Once the game is over the Giant is untied from his Bouncy Shackles and the Hoppers can then be used by the kids!*

124. *The Giant (*and his helper) has set it such you only escape when your name is called and so...*

125. *I have seen ** his list so wait till I call your name...*

126. *Call out the birthday boy first, then in order the smallest to the biggest so no body crashing occurs.*

127. *You don't really ** need read from a list here as you should know the invitees by name*

128. *Or failing this you can just point to whoever*

129. *I have never needed help any child, as the pull to get his/her ice cream, **no matter what,** is too great!*

130. *And to encourage him/her get the group to chant his/her name*

131. *"Go Jenny/Jude/Jeremy or whoever!"*

The beauty of using small sweets is that you get a lot in a bag full and just like the larger than required amount of tennis balls, both can be used to put in the post birthday goody bags!

↑ OFF YOU GO TRY ME ↑

IF YOU THINK

YOU'VE GOT THE METTLE?

But now for the Mother/Child Sweet Baking Bond

7 CHRISTMAS MYA'S CAKE (Part 1 of 2) BAKING

So here goes nothing, hoping the kids don't make too much of a mess!? <> That is if they want to help?!

- **1st:-** *a few days beforehand, pre-soak your choice of fruit ↓# in the liqueur/alcohol of your choice ↓# <u>turning over each morning</u>*

<u>BUT ON THE DAY BEFORE ALL THE MIXING ETC TAKES PLACE – THERE ARE CERTAIN IMPORTANT TASKS:-</u> Pictures are added at the end for reference – *especially the tin lining process!*

A. The type of circular baking tin (here 9in) to use showing its removable base and retaining clip...

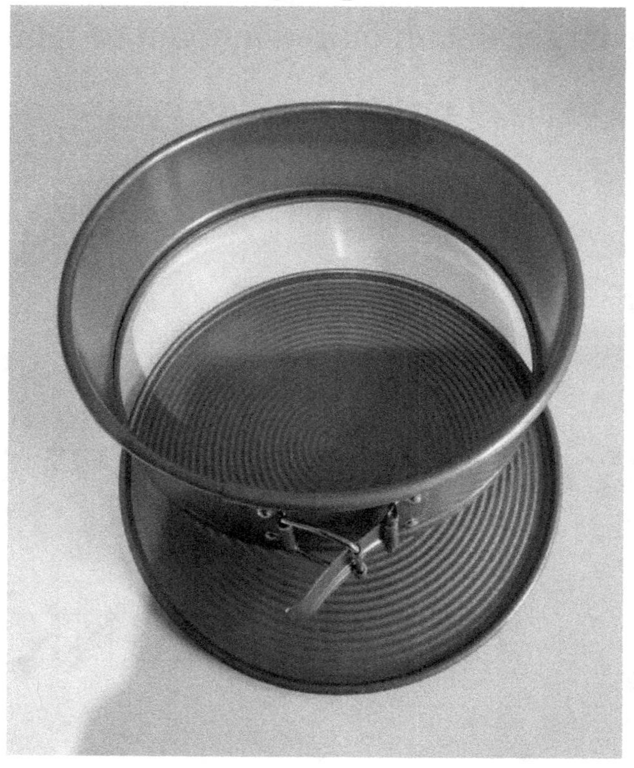

B. The base extracted...

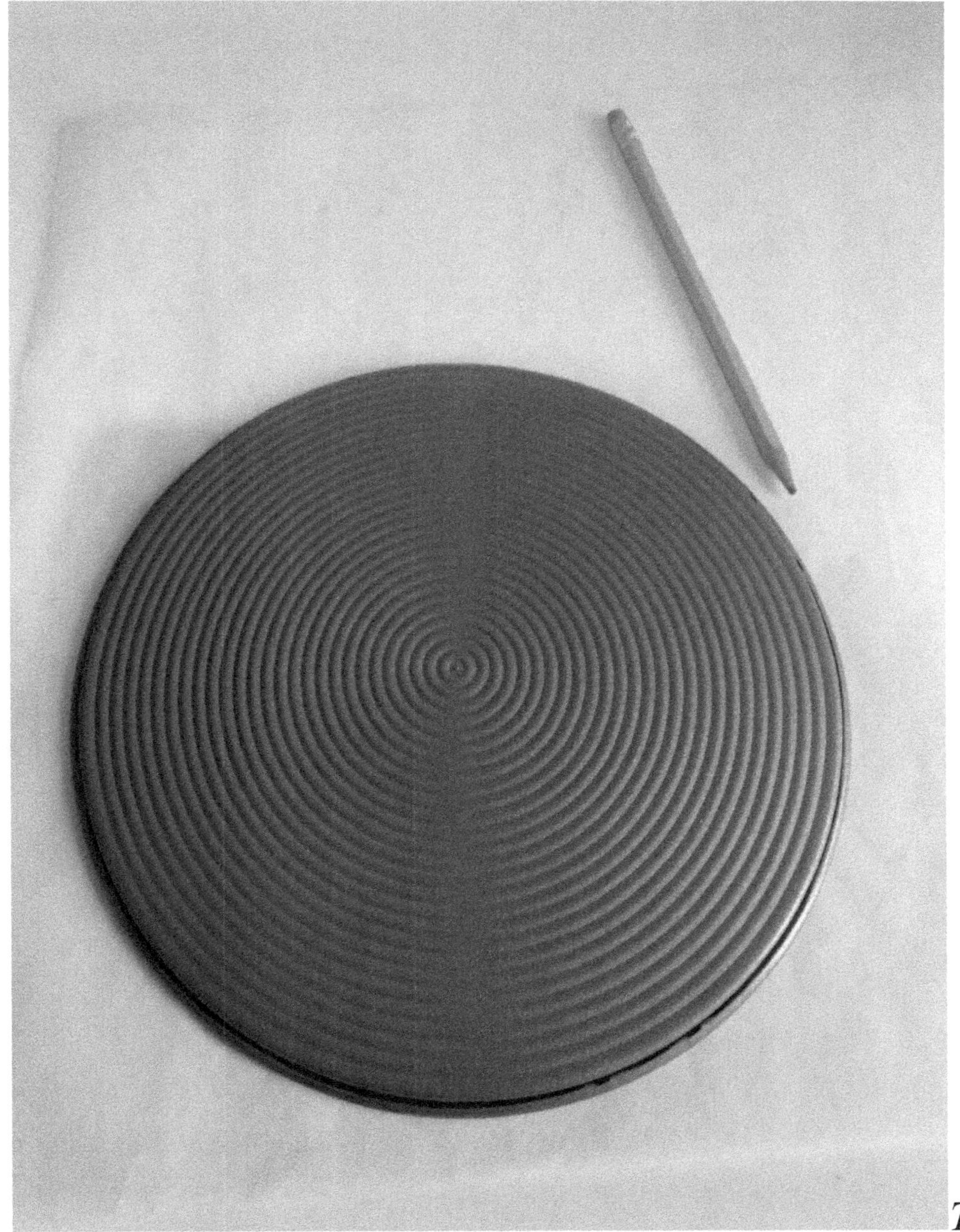

The photo shows it placed on the baking paper ready to cut 2 impressions as instructed above...then comes the inner surround cuts..

C. The far end ↓ is folded over about ¾ inch and cut diagonally...

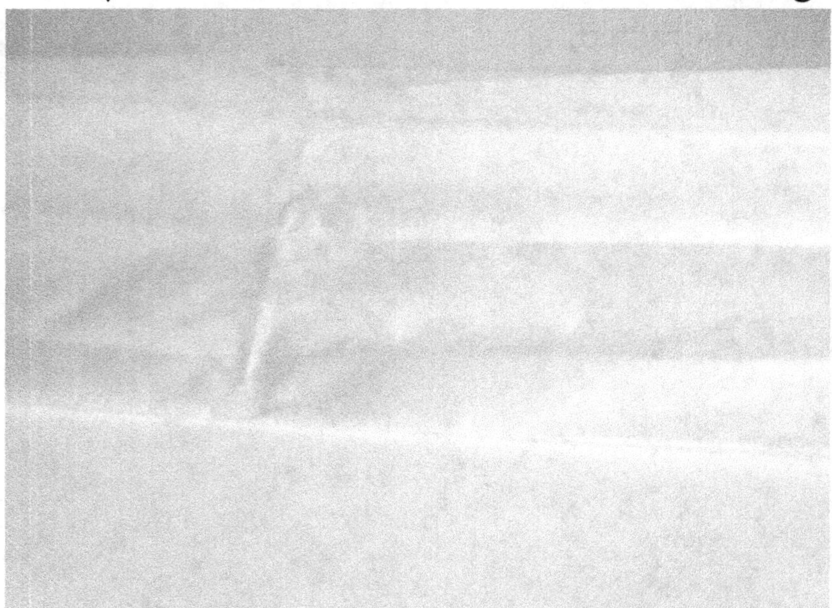

D. Here the diagonal cutting exercise...

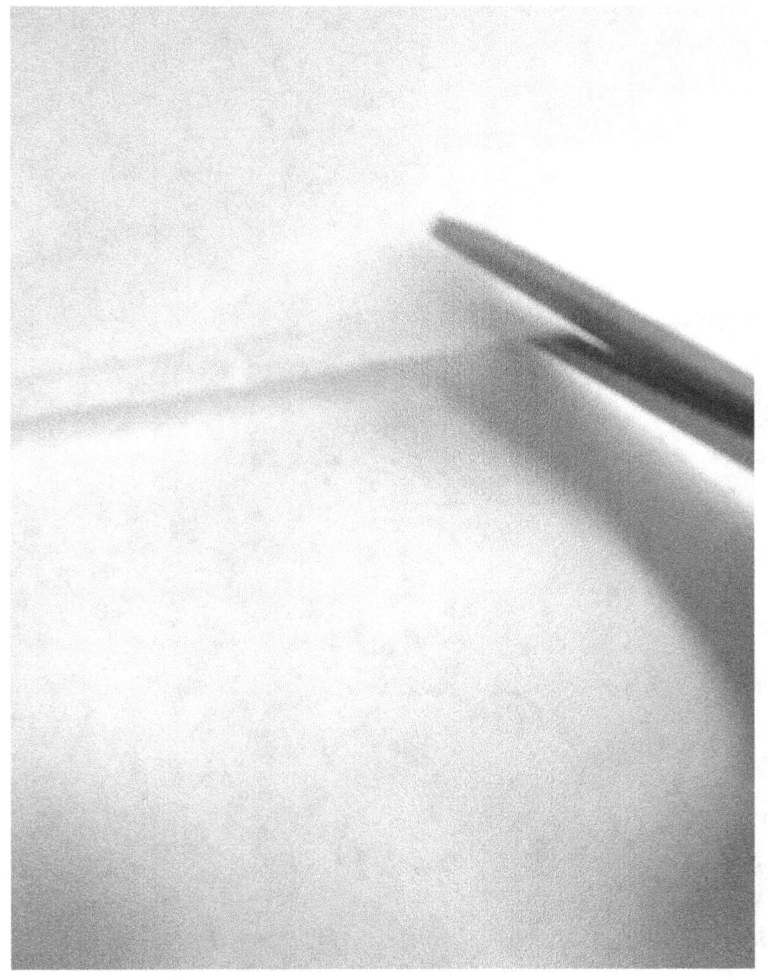

E. The hem pre-cut, then it will be easy to insert without creasing...

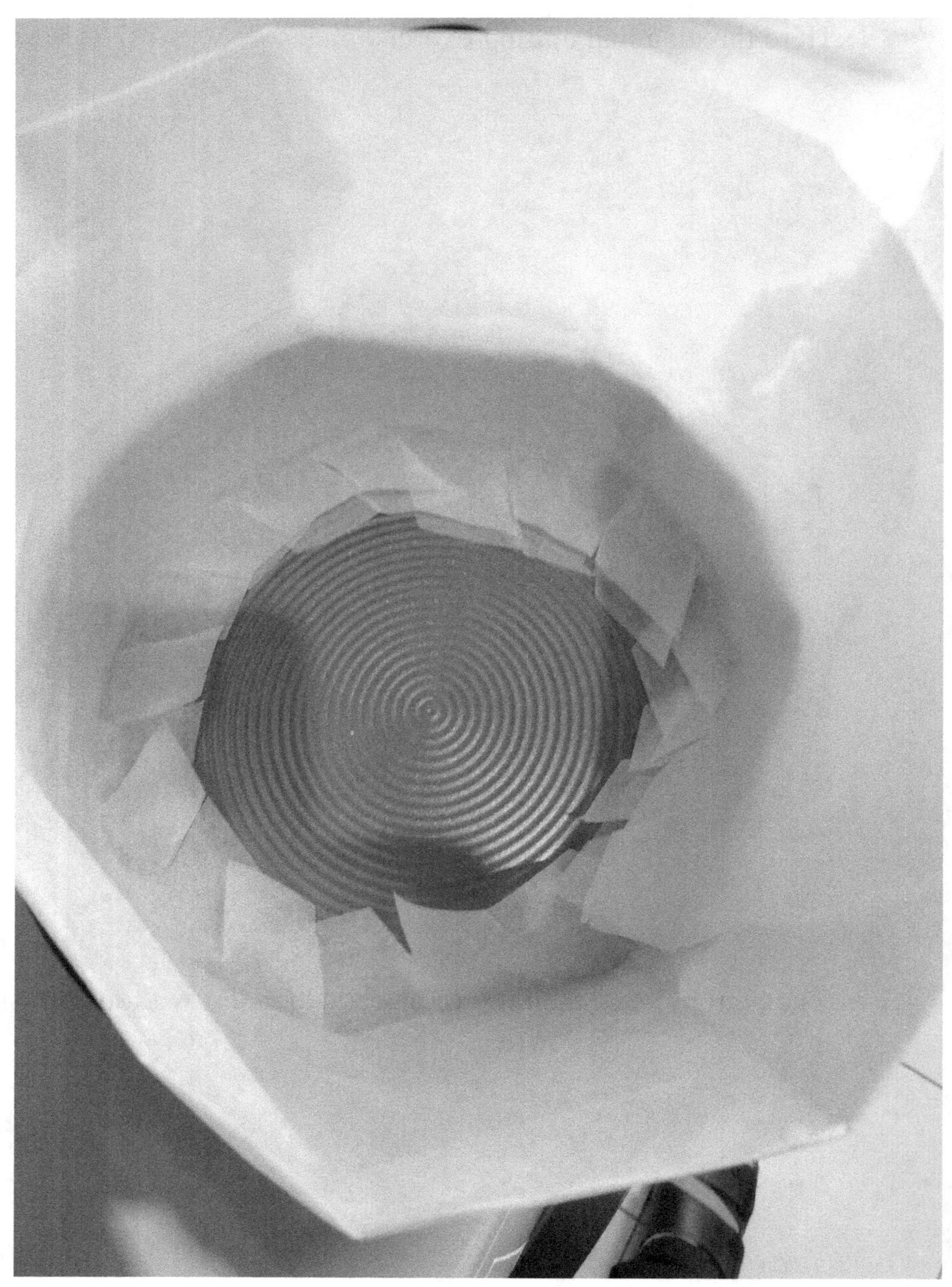

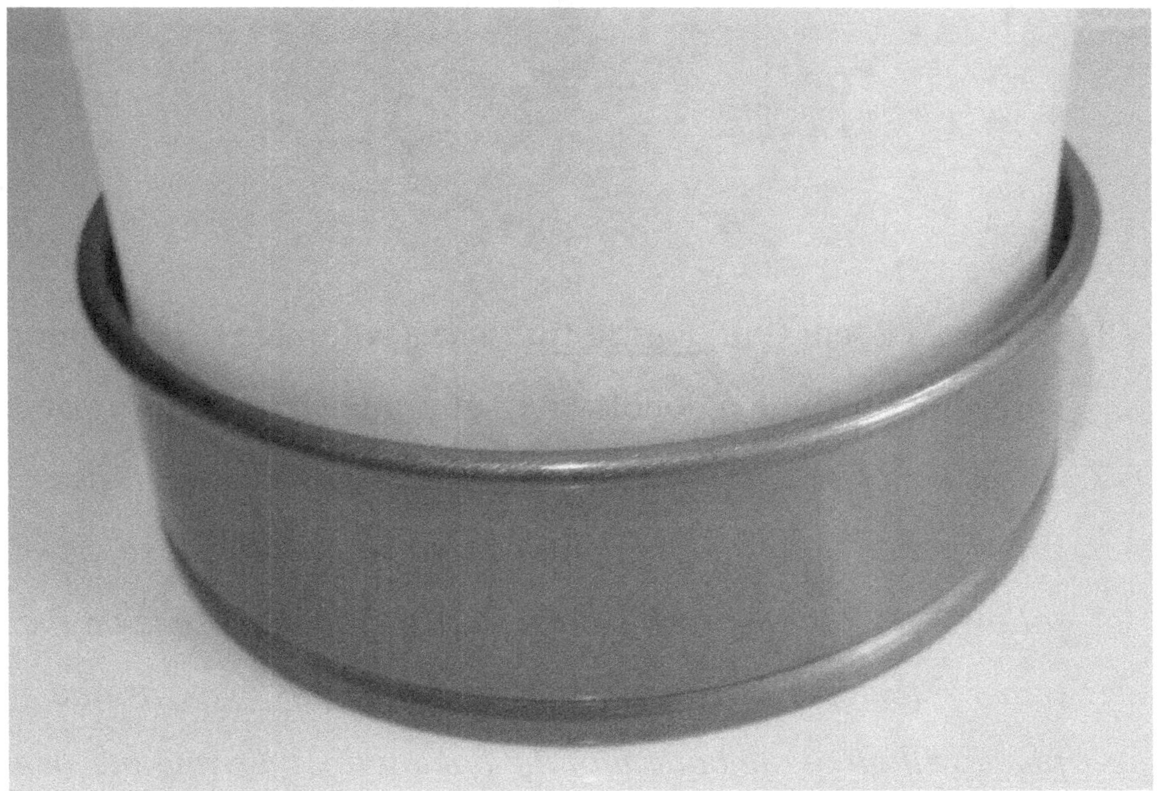

For me, perhaps not you: The inner is not too high as it allows the
cake to rise, but additionally the greaseproof paper will be used
after baking to fold over + store.

<u>So remember to bake on the bottom shelf
with nothing else!</u>

NOW

G. All the greaseproof/baking paper to be additionally greased
using such as...

1. **Grease** a 23cm (9in) **<u>round tin</u>** I use a soft margarine/buttery ↓ spread & line with a double layer of pre-cut greaseproof paper -

2. *... the knack to a lining a well-greased cake tin with grease-proof paper is the shaping/cutting and not just the base as follows: lay the removable base from the tin and place on the paper – then pencil around and cut but <u>do this twice</u> as one piece will go at the bottom of the baking tin, then another over the inner surround... Picture assistance above.*

3. *Before the inner tin lining, you need run a tape measure around the tin to determine its circumference, then add a couple more inches; cut your greaseproof paper to this length; fold exactly in two lengthways. Picture assistance above.*

4. *With the inner surround there is a knack-trick: at the end where the 2 ends meet, fold the bottom over giving it an inch hem; then make regular diagonal ¾ cuts at every inch along the whole length of the hemmed paper; this cut hem will then be easy to fold onto the base of the tin where the 1ˢᵗ greased circular paper is laid; then with the 2nd pre-cut paper on top. Picture assistance above.*

5. *All paper to be additionally greased using the same* soft ↑ *above* margarine/buttery spread *before placing in the tin, so all stick together and don't allow any mix to escape…*

6. *Although not part of the ingredients – keep pack of ground almonds handy if the mix gets too runny (Below)*

After this initial set up you can let the children get involved wherever you/they feel comfortable – their involvement both shows them how to bake and the work needed beforehand/after and for them the 'after' licking the mixing bowl its blades &/or spoon/spatula dry!

1. Preheat the oven to 140c (120c fan) = (gas 1)
2. And here you can roast (4oz) crunched up almonds (See Later)
3. Take out your 9oz of butter to soften up (See Later)

•••••••••••••••

- This recipe contains at least a kilo of fruit!
- And so
- Some electric mixers/bowls might not be large enough!
- Mine is 9in wide x 6in high. And so
- You can use just half: the other ingredients will remain the same
- Or you can make two cakes: although the other ingredients will remain the same you'll have to do the job twice! And so
- Or you can adapt as described later (Mixing In ↓)

•••••••••••••••

>>>> The Ingredients...

- I like to chop and change! And so
- I will give alternatives as I go along!

- *175 g (6oz) raisins#*
- *500g (12oz) currants#*
- *350g (12oz) sultans#*
- *# # # Or you could also just get a 1kilo pack of mixed fruit – but, care, as I prefer my raisins pipless!   And so*
- *I prefer the Waitrose Italian Vine Mix*

- *# And* alternatives *so here are mine...*
- *# Instead of usual brandy/cognac try to soak all fruit in any sweet liqueur (half a large bottle at least)(undiluted), or even coffee flavoured Tia Maria, even Bailey's, or even Rum Malibu, or a bottle of ginger wine which is great too!)*
- *# As above ensure soak for at least a few days so all the booze is absorbed.*
- *# Making sure you mix/stir daily.*
- *# When ready sieve over a jug – keep the excess liquor* [XX].
- *# This you retain for future use adding to cake after left to stand*

- 250g (10oz) glace cherries, but these need attention! *And so*
- *Cut the cherries first, then wash them, then place them in the prepared bowl of flour mix (see later ↓) – in this way they won't sink whilst the cake rises (if you cut them after washing you'll still get that sticky/gooey mess in the mix*

- Finely grate zest of 2 large oranges & a few oz of mixed peel ~
- *~ Here I improvise to use other similar ingredients! And so*
- *~ Instead try using the contents of those old half empty jam jars*

- *~ I'm sure you'll also find an old half empty marmalade one!*
- *~ Additionally/or cut up any uneaten dried fruit! (e.g. apricots)*

- 250g (9oz) butter – Many recipes fail to mention the following: *Ensure you leave it out in warm kitchen to soften up (above); Then cut into about 9, even 18 pieces so you can add gradually.*
- 250g (9oz) light muscovado (brown) sugar, *or golden caster.*
- 4 large eggs – I like to prepare mine beforehand - *And so*
- *Break them up, put all in one cup/jug and stir together - ready to pour into the mix –(Picture Below)*

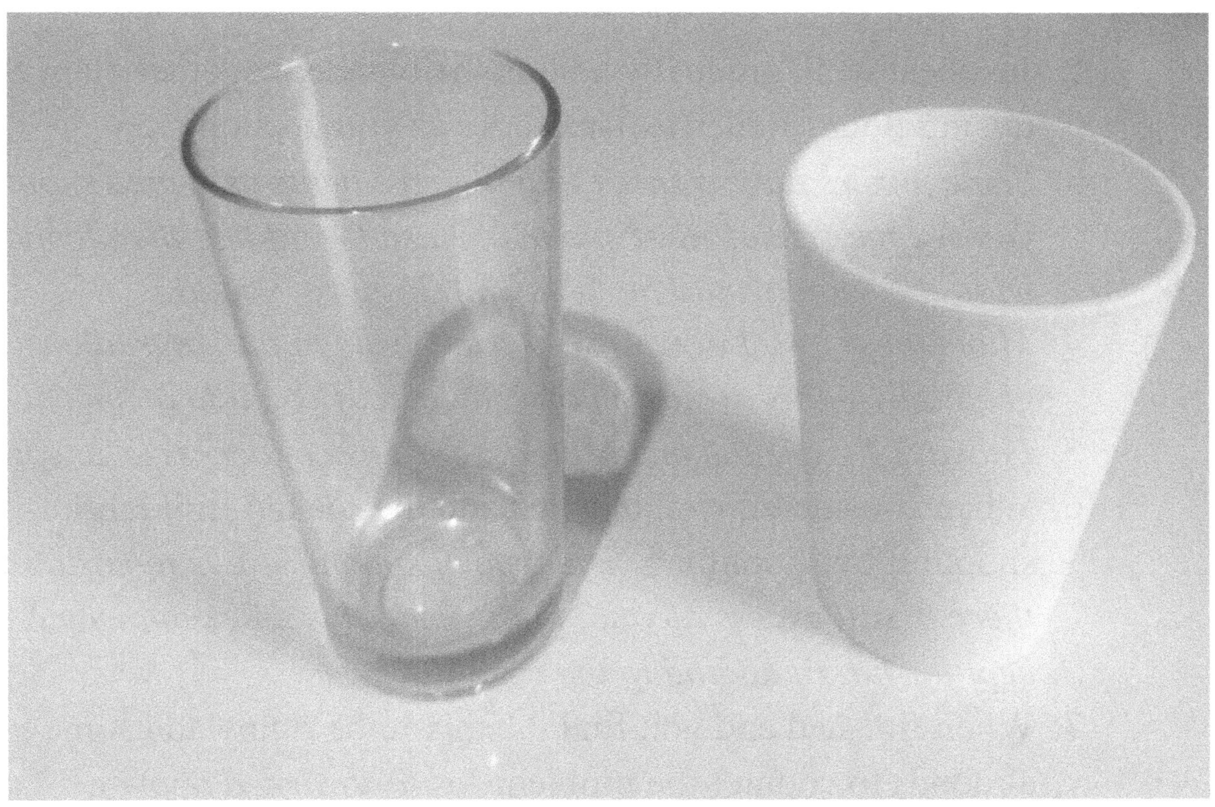

- 1 tablespoon of black treacle – I am not a lover of this! *And so*
- *Use golden syrup (perhaps Maple flavoured); even honey!*
- 100g (4oz) blanched almonds – *chop/break up when at home – and <u>roast for 15 minutes in the preheating oven</u> (as above) - although have you also then considered adding the crunch of poppy seeds?*
- 75g (3oz) self-raising flour

- 175g (6oz) plain flour *And so*
- *Place both batches of flour in one bowl & add in the cherries* ↑
- 1½ tsp mixed spice

....

THE MIXING

1. Add the butter, sugar, peels, treacle/syrup, almonds, mixed spices into your mixing bowl.
2. Just beat well, gradually adding the blended together plain & self-raising flour (+ cherries) and eggs as you go along...
3. *Some mixers have a shoot to add ingredients as it mixes, but if you see the size of sieve spoon [XX] I use for adding the alcoholic fruit, the spout would be too small. Picture 9 below...*
4. *Mine doesn't so I always stop * the cycle to add ingredients gradually – this avoids a possible mess if you add at speed!*
5. *I always * raise the mixer blades for ease of access – no spilling.*
6. When considered well blended add the soaked fruit large spoonful by spoonful [XX] *The type of spoon I use is to ensure if there is still excess alcohol in the fruit, this will run away & to be kept for future adding to the cake flavour!*
7. When finished and you find the mix to be runny add some ground almonds to counter the problem *(as forewarned above)*.
8. When ready, carefully pour into the prepared lined cake tin and level off. The kids can then be allowed to clean the mixing bowl dry with finger &/or spatula &/or spoon! And perhaps you can focus on the cake mix laden mixer blades!?
9. Bake in the centre of oven for 4 hours *, or until cake feels firm to the touch: it should be a rich golden brown AND a heated skewer comes out clean.

10. During cooking the cake s/b covered with brown paper *(not greaseproof paper which is too light and can be blown away in fan ovens)* (The paper is there to avoid the top being burnt if the mix is exposed to heat for too long). *

11. And * s/b removed an hour or so before it is due to be finished.

12. Test every 20 minutes thereafter with a hot skewer:- if it comes out dry then switch off oven.

13. Likely as not it will the colder part of the year...so leave the oven door ajar to warm up your kitchen work area...

BUT IT YOU WANT SOMETHING SIMPLER – HERE IS MY

8 CAKE BAKING SIMPLE MYA MINGLING MAKING

<u>WARNING</u> - ANYONE WITH A NUT ALLERGY, OR INTOLERANCE* TO ANY OF THE XMAS CAKE INGREDIENTS BEFORE, *SHOULD NOT HELP OUT THERE,* BUT, RATHER BE INVOLVED WITH A MORE SIMPLE CAKE LIKE A MADEIRA >>

*** NB Celiacs (Gluten Free) + Dairy Free - again should use substitutes for any to which they are intolerant ↓**

- 175G/6OZ SOFTENED BUTTER
- 175G/6OZ CASTER SUGAR
- 3 LARGE EGGS
- 250G/9OZ SELF-RAISING FLOUR
- LEMON ZEST (OPTIONAL#)
- 2-3 TABLESPOONS OF MILK ##

Whilst making the cake mix preheat the oven to 170°C, gas mark 3 (Fan = 150°C)

Butter your medium sized cake tin and line with greaseproof paper.

Mix/Whisk the butter, sugar (# + lemon zest) in a large bowl until fluffy.

Continue whisking, slowly adding add one egg at a time, then, again slowly, the flour. ## Add milk if mixture gets/looks too dry)

Pour mix into your cake tin & **then it is kiddies spatula/bowl licking time!**

(Although for their non-lazy responsible upbringing -
Should they not be made to help wash/dry/clear up afterwards!?)

Bake at temperature of 170C for 45 minutes until golden and springy and a (warmed) skewer comes out clean.

PS If the cake is browning too quickly, loosely cover the top with foil, but remember to remove it shortly before the end of cooking.

Sit the cake tin on a wire rack and leave for 15 minutes.

 # For The Zing/Zest In The Cake <> Rather Than Freeze It Get The Kids To Help You Ice It Later After It Has Cooled Down – They'll Love To Help <u>Again</u> If Only To Lick The Spatula Dry!

NB If un-iced you can leave for a day or so – No worries as it freezes well.

<u>(Wrap in Foil).</u>

>>>

<u>BUT NOW IT IS BACK TO THE GREAT OUTDOORS FOR A LARGE GATHERING AND ALL THE GAME COMBINATIONS IT HOLDS WITHIN/WITHOUT???!!!</u>

>>>

9 SOCIAL GATHERING YOUNG & OLD PRIZE MIXES!

....

THE EXPANDED TITLE OF THIS CHAPTER IS
<u>INDOOR/OUTDOOR MIXED PARTY</u>
<u>YOUNG & OLD MINGLING TIME</u>
<u>WIN AND YOU GET FED FIRST!</u>

<u>AND IT IS ANOTHER</u>

<u>MAMMOTH PREPARED PRESENTATION</u>

<u>ADULT TIME</u>

I HAVE NEVER BEEN ENAMOURED OF THE

CONVENTIONAL SEATING PLAN WHERE, FOR EXAMPLE,

AT A CELEBRATORY GATHERING, THERE ARE 9 COUPLES

AT A RESTAURANT AROUND A LARGE EXTENDED TABLE

SITTING AND THE HUSBAND & WIFE WOULD ALWAYS BE

NEXT TO EACH OTHER

– "WHAT WOULD THEY HAVE MORE TO TALK ABOUT,

BEING CONTINUALLY IN EACH OTHER'S PROXIMITY ALL

THEIR LIFE?"

AND THERE AGAIN, AS WITH MOST HUSBANDS THERE WAS ALSO THE INHIBITING FACTOR OF BEING WITHIN EARSHOT OF THE *WIFE!*

And this is also what trying to avoid that now new notorious Covid flu type killer has taught us is how difficult it is for the majority being in one's partner's, or family's pocket for too long – as tempers can fray etc!!

All the time would be an impossibility for so many!

For me, when entertaining, it was not a problem, though perhaps challenging for some, who always seemed to be only inches from their spouse.

But they eventually came round as their embarrassment fear of being the odd ones out would always win out in the end!

And winning with another person was a novel if not somewhat a new invigorating experience, if not just to have a different point of view coming from their new game partner source!

But, back to my restaurant, celebrating my birthday, anniversary, for example, or whatever, I would insist that the male move 3 places to the right before each of four courses; thus, ensuring someone new to chat with as the meal was consumed – it played havoc with the waiters remembering who ordered what!

But that was all part of <u>my</u> *mad*(dening) & *crazy,* fun filled, mind!

But, not as maddening if you had to win a game to get the meal you were after!

<u>Confused</u>?

You won't be after you've read the next session >>>>

For some reason I tend to favour the kids, not the adults, at events, which older/old fashioned (?) people believe children should be seen, but not heard.

Well, here they were the centre of it all, and their word was the law this time!

But, I won't ask you to go to extremes in their home life book: so no building wooden castles from scratch – that goes on your back burner of things to do to entertain your brood, especially if it incorporates steps up & slides down, large enough to accommodate them, plus their friends, in the back garden!

Imagine catering in the back garden for the same 18 restaurant attendees, plus, say, two under elevens (boys &/or girls) thrown in for good measure, how to get the kids involved & kill their boredom?

Arrange **(1)** couple's games and **(2)** games between the sexes.
For both, the host & hostess are the quizmaster & adjudicator; for the first, the kids, the helpers/judges; for the second participants.

But, first a mug of soup in the garden: always being different, I would baulk at the idea of just one flavour: so it would be half a dozen assorted cartons into one large pot and served up as a *'flavoured concoction!* Oddly enough, all seem to enjoy the *mix*, although some are totally/blissfully unaware.

NB *Once again I'd be aware of any food allergies/intolerances!*

....

Now follows the simple pre-food initial ice-breaker >>>

For (1) there will be 8 mixed couples *(i.e. not husband & wife – as I said above)* seated together in a large circle facing each other.
You will then need: 8 pens and pads, a ruler, *a step ladder*, 18 pairs of shoes!
A *'Get to know you'* quiz then takes place with such questions as:
- *Write how many of the contestants have brown eyes* (see how each hides their colour from the others);
- Write how many are natural blondes;
- Write the ages of each, including the hosts;
- Write a list of who (in their slippers) is the tallest to the shortest man/woman/all*;
- Write whose pair of shoes are these*;
- Write what size are they (including ½ sizes).

The list is limitless.

A point for each correct answer.

OFF YOU GO TRY ME

And the children's involvement?

*This is where the kids come in:

- For the shoes you make sure everyone brings their slippers and leaves their shoes at the front door and at the prescribed moment the children randomly bring each pair in turn, one or two causing them to hold their noses because of a supposed smell, to be assessed/guessed;

- For the shortest/tallest lists there will be disputes, so people might need be measured up against each other with the kids on the step ladder with their rulers making the decision here;

- Then at the end, the top scoring couple, then the second and so on, would be led into the house in order to where the food was laid;

- IN THIS WAY THE BEST SCORERS WOULD GET FIRST PICK OF THE FOOD/DRINK (<u>THE CHILDREN WOULD ALREADY HAVE THEIRS READY</u>).

THE HOST/HOSTESS WILL HAVE LAID THE HOT &/OR COLD BUFFET INSIDE WELL BEFORE, WITH NO REAL PRIOR PLANNING OF WHO LIKES WHAT AS WINNING HERE GETS YOU TO THE FRONT OF THE QUEUE!

(ALLERGY SUFFERERS EXCLUDED)

(AS THEY HAVE BEEN SPECIALLY CATERED FOR)

>>>>>>>>>>

Now follows the major pre-dessert goodies Male v Female Competition >>>

With (No.2), the games between the sexes the kids would also take their integral part. (If you only have the same sex kids present, then you need decide who joins which team).

There will be 2 teams, with respective captains. You will then need:

- 1 pen and pad;
- 3 jigsaw puzzles (one each of 25, 50 & 100 pieces) for completion; 1st
- 3 small Lego toys to put together; 1st
- From floor level, the tallest Jenga to stack, but one brick upon another, not structured as in the box; 2nd
- One simple 40 clued crossword; 1st
- A simple (tie-breaking) quiz like preparing a list of the _different_ * names of 12 of our Kings/Queens – (Including spouses – Henry 8th had 7!) since William the Conqueror. (* i.e. Queen Elizabeth 1st and Queen Elizabeth 2nd, would only count as one)
- The winning tie-break team would be the one who best matched the Host/Hostess pre-prepared list secreted in a sealed envelope - the kids would do the cross checking!

OFF YOU GO TRY ME

All this going on with a half hour time limit – view the ensuing panic, deciding who does what, and when those who have completed their task mucks in with the others still struggling!

HOW COME?

[1st] **Simply, that when each task is completed**
> **it is 10 points to the first to finish, nil for the 2nd!**

NB *Care when judging if the Lego task is performed totally correctly as it has been known that the head of the lorry driver was facing the wrong way yet still fooled the Judge!*

[2nd] **The Jenga Tower is judged/measured more than once during the contest by the Host, as it as likely it will be found that the opposition have managed to make theirs taller in the interim.**

No jealous kid (young or old) knocking the opponent's one over:-

**Or simply say there will be a 10 point penalty – then he/she will understand!**

....

The scoring for each individually determined, say 10, except the crossword where there's a point for each correct word solution.

OFF YOU GO TRY ME – I KNOW YOU _**LADIES**_ WANT TO!

THE WINNING TEAM HAS FIRST DIBS AT THE CAKE SURPRISES: SOMETHING LIKE ~~THIS~~ MINE – WOW!

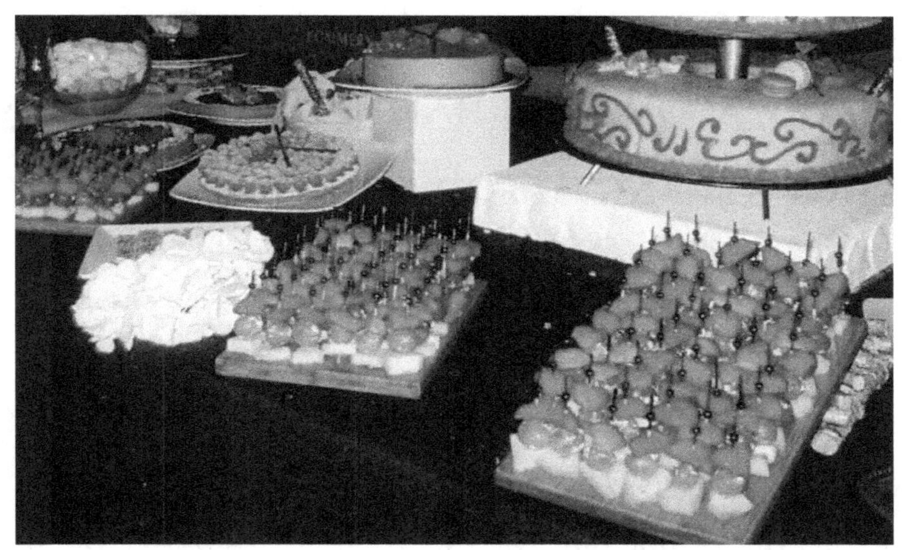

....

10 A TEST OF STRENGTH FOR LADIES EYES ONLY

>>> ↓↓↓

Something only for the woman (trusting the men haven't read this also!) to start with, the (5) scattered bricks (see below) a test of strength where the ladies win (as the Hostess arranges for the solution ## to be given them beforehand)!

Solution >>> http://www.magictricktips.com/magictricktips05.php
Game entitled:

'Women are truly the stronger Race!'

Nominate one person from each team to pick up the 5 bricks with one hand, in one go, (the other behind the back) and place them on the table in front of you.

Make the man go first and allow him 30 seconds: his female is asked to leave in the meantime *(where she is shown the answer).* She returns when the time has elapsed, then she does her stuff.

Quickest time wins. I will eat my hat if the fellas know the solution, so are bound to lose! Women Rule! And don't we deserve too?

SO FOR LADIES EYES ONLY >>> ↑↑↑

....

11 A GROUP HELLO - WHO ARE YOU AGAIN?

We have recently been entertaining the family without the kids around to cause distraction, as they always do, and to just give you more than a glimpse of what this Book contains, here are some of the various game types, John & I have employed in past times, to keep all the Adults of varying abilities focused – and at times it is some task to get the balance spot on?!

(Further variations of the following themes appear in the Book).

1) HELLO! WHO ARE YOU AGAIN?

a. So here you are with your party guests, friends AND relatives, placed in the garden area, so they won't see what you have prepared, with their teas & coffees in hand, idly chatting. But, and it is my usual Big But how much do they really know about each other.

b. And here, as some monopolise conversations with others, often the timid sort, find themselves unheard, here all MUST take their turn to participate in front of ALL!

c. The subsequent *'I didn't know that!'* conversations will neatly glide into the next session...

d. Here is my sample *'Getting to Know You Better'* Quiz Questionnaire for the guests excluding the *Host – who will still be in the middle of so many more preparations (later)...

e. Here, for ease, there are 4 Principals:- Norah/Ken/Bob & Babs...

No.	A Tick for Each Correct Answer Excluding 21 & 22 – Where Nearest Wins – Answers Below ↓	
1.	Borough You Live In Bob?	
2.	Borough You Live In Norah?	
3.	Borough You Live In Ken?	
4.	Borough You Live In Babs?	
5.	Whose is the Biggest Shoe Size	
6.	Name Those with Blue Eyes	
7.	Name All Those Left handers	
8.	*Inc. Michael Who's the Oldest	
9.	Nearest Tube/Subway Station to Bob	
10.	Nearest Tube/Subway Station to Norah	
11.	Nearest Tube/Subway Station to Ken	
12.	Nearest Tube/Subway Station to Babs	
13.	Norah's Favourite Football Team	
14.	Bob's Favourite Football Team	
15.	Ken's Favourite Football Team	
16.	Bab's Favourite Football Team	
17.	Bab's Favourite Holiday destination	
18.	Bob's Favourite Holiday destination	

		Total Correct Ticks	
19.	Norah's Favourite Holiday destination	
20.	Ken's Favourite Holiday destination	
21.	Total Number of Siblings that You ALL have?	
22.	The total of all your 4 ages	
23.	What's more: combined ages of Bob/Ken, or Norah/Barbara?	
24.	Bab's Favourite Pop Star?	
25.	Bob's Favourite Pop Star?	
26.	Ken's Favourite Pop Star?	
27.	Norah's Favourite Pop Star?	
28.	Norah's Favourite Pop Group?	
29.	Ken's Favourite Pop Group?	
30.	Bob's Favourite Pop Group?	
31.	Bab's Favourite Pop Group?	
32.	Who's Left Footed?	
	Total Correct Ticks	
Now I hope you know so much more about Each Other		

This breaks the ice and also get people out of their shell, if they hadn't already during the initial/opening tea/coffee chit chat session.

*The question combinations are endless – they work best when so many are the * Host's friends who are not that well known to all...AND this hopefully makes each now more well known to the others!*

HERE IS A SURPRISE ONE YOU'VE NEVER ENCOUNTERED

12 A GROUP HELLO - WHAT ARE YOU AGAIN?

ROUND 2 WHAT AM I EATING? <>

One Point Per Answer <>

Here Norah the Hostess has laid a grand spread before her contesting guests <>

All they have to do is eat/enjoy AND answer questions of what is laid before them <>

1. *Which* fish is in breadcrumbs?	
2. Which ordinary cheese is in the Cheese Straws?	
3. Flatback Crackers are Olive & ??? Flavour	
4. The Horseradish flavour is ????	
5. What are the two	
6. flavour ingredients of The Chutneys	
7. Norah's jam is raspberry but yours is elderflower and ??	
8. Norah has her plain crisps but what flavour is the other before you??	

9. What are the 3 main	
10. Bread Dipper	
11. Flavours	
12. Is the butter on Norah's plate salted or unsalted? (No tasting!)	
13. Which Fruit is covered in Dark Chocolate?	
(You can answer in English) (The song) 14. What did people do on the Avignon Bridge	<u>They???</u>
15. On which River does it stand	
16. Translate into English the *Neuf* in Chateau Neuf du Pape	
17. Before she brings back the Chateau Neuf du Pape <> Its Proof is ?? Nearest Wins.	
18. How many pieces of fish as in Qu1 were originally laid before you, before you ate them all?	

I trust you get my Food/Drink Competition Drift?

The Food & Drink Types are Boundless – My Samples Above

Note: The Scampi question is purposely No 1 on the list, because all will start sampling it to guess it...and you'll notice the follow up is No 18 by which time all the evidence will have been eaten and the number set out beforehand, forgotten?!

13 XMAS CAKE MAKING INNER SECRETS REVEALED

Round 3 *That ubiquitous Christmas Cake re-appears – a sample was part of the opening Buffet Rounds 1-2 - So here simply the guests have to guess the ingredients <>*

No.	*My Xmas Cake recipe in this Book has mostly has the same ingredients and made the same way! <> Here For the Guest's Guess – A Point for Each Correct - ↓*	
1.	700, 800, 900, 1000 gr of fruit?	
2.	100, 200 or 300 gr of almonds?	
3.	What is the crunchy nut inside?	
4.	500ml, 600ml, 700ml alcohol?	
5.	15% 20% 25% 30% 40% proof	
6.	7, 8, 9 or 10 oz of butter?	
7.	100, 200, 250, 0r 350gr sugar?	
8.	4, 5, 6 or 7 eggs?	
9.	7, 8 or 9 inch baking tin?	
10.	3, 4, 5 or 6 oz s/raising flour?	
11.	3, 4, 5 or 6 oz plain flour?	
12.	120, 130, 140c oven heat?	
13.	2½, 3, 4, 4½ cooking time?	
14.	What's my jam substitute for mixed peel	
15.	Eggs medium or large?	
16.	Fruit used Raisins/Currants & ?	
17.	No. marzipan slabs to cover cake?	
18.	No. icing packets to cover cake?	
19.	3 Spices used Ginger/nutmeg and ?	
20.	Month Xmas cake prep started?	
	Total Correct Ticks	

AND SO BACK IN THE GARDEN >>>

14 GARDENING CAN BE FUN BUT THE SPELLING NEVER

<ins>Round 4 GARDEN FLOWER TIME x The Clock 10 MINUTES</ins>
<ins>It is usual that so many of the Older generation spend more time</ins>
<ins>in their Gardens: they know the name, but can they spell it?</ins>

No.	Gardener's Questions	Answers
	Correct My Spelling ↓	
1.	Pairrennial (Not an Annual)	
2.	Pestemon	
3.	Achellia	
4.	Cracosmea	
5.	Delfinnium	
6.	Eringiun	
7.	Youforbea	
8.	Jeranum	
9.	Heycherea	
10.	Anoneme	
11.	Popover (A Poppy)	
12.	Pramoola	
13.	(Sleep Time) Hybornate	
14.	(Non woody stems) Hurbaseos	
	↓ Does it Like Ericaceous Soil?	↓ Y or N ↓
15.	Azalea	Y or N
16.	Acer	Y or N
17.	Pieris	Y or N
18.	Is Rhododendron Ponticum invasive?	Y or N
19.	Are monkshood & wolfsbane the same	Y or N
20.	Are monkshood & wolfsbane poisonous	↑ Y or N ↑
	TOTAL >>>	

HERE ARE THE ANSWERS FOR YOU…

ANSWERS TO ROUND 4 FLOWER TIME

No.	Gardener's Questions	Answers
	Correct My Spelling ↓	
1.	Pairrennial (Not an Annual)	Perennial
2.	Pestemon	Penstemon
3.	Achellia	Achillea
4.	Cracosmea	Crocosmia
5.	Delfinnium	Delphinium
6.	Eringiun	Eryngium
7.	Youforbea	Euphorbia
8.	Jeranum	Geranium
9.	Heycherea	Heuchera
10.	Anoneme	Anemone
11.	Popover (A Poppy)	Papaver
12.	Pramoola	Primula
13.	(Sleep Time) Hybornate	Hibernate
14.	(Non woody stems) Hurbaseos	Herbaceous
	↓ Does it Like Ericaceous Soil?	
15.	Azalea	Yes
16.	Acer	Yes
17.	Pieris	Yes
18.	Is Rhododendron Ponticum invasive?	Yes
19.	Are monkshood & wolfsbane the same	Yes = Aconitum
20.	Are monkshood & wolfsbane poisonous	Yes = Aconitum

15 BRIDGE A GAP A TRAVEL GAMBLE INTERLUDE (with answers)

A linked prelude to the next 2 Games!　　*

No.	Question	Answers
1.	**Bridge suits ranking downward in order are** *	spades, hearts, diamonds, clubs >>>
2.	No. of Points below the line to win?	100
3.	Bullet is slang for which card	Ace
4.	Is Devil's Coup OR Devil's Grip a Bridge Tactic?	Coup – the other is from Solitaire
<	*In Which Country are these...*	
5.	Great Belt Bridge	Denmark
6.	Chapel Bridge (Wooden/Covered)	Switzerland
7.	Chengyang Bridge	China
8.	Brooklyn Bridge	USA
9.	Alcantara Bridge	Spain
10.	Si-o-se Pol made of 33 arches	Iran
11.	Akashi-Kaikyo Bridge	Japan
12.	Rialto Bridge	Italy
13.	Charles Bridge	Czech Republic
14.	Millau Bridge	France
15.	Golden Gate Bridge	USA
16.	Ponte Vecchio	Italy
17.	London Bridge	USA
18.	Indonesian businessman **Michael Bambang Hartono** (net worth $18.4 billion) is one of the most successful of the bridge-playing billionaires, winning medals in three world championships. Gold Silver or Bronze?	**Bronze**
19.	My Michael met Victoria Coren Mitchell a couple of times & discussed tactics: Which is her favourite money making card game forté?	**Poker**
20.	The next year 2004 was she 1st, 2nd, or 3rd in a European Championship	2nd

**THE NEXT ASSORTMENT WILL AS LIKELY ALL BE
INDOORS WHERE THE GAMBLING/COMPETITVE
EXPERIENCE ELEMENT WILL COME TO THE FORE
AND HERE ARRANGE TEAMS AS PAIRS
ie 6 PEOPLE = THREE TEAMS OF 2!**

**BUT HERE WE NEED INTRODUCE SOMETHING NEW AND
ADDITIONAL A SCREEN DIVIDING SYSTEM TO ENSURE
NO CHEATING >>.**

<u>**PS**</u> *Regarding the Dividers mentioned above...*

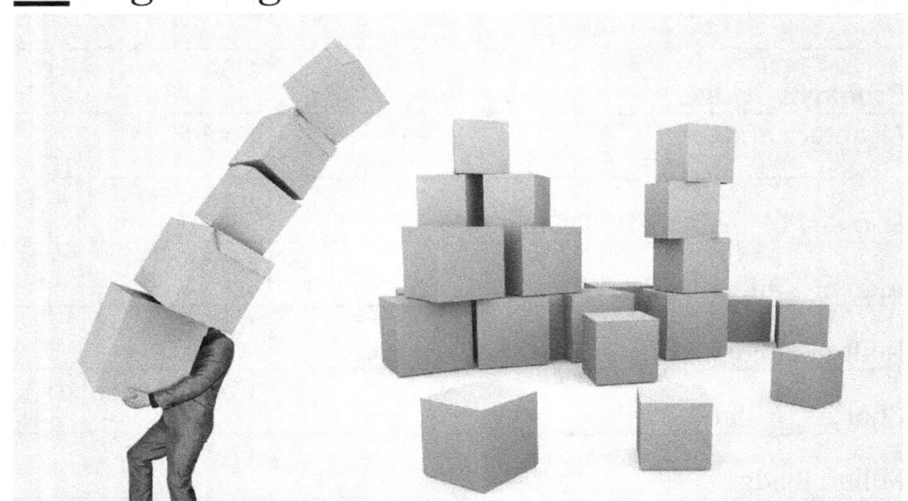

<u>Many Juggling Thanks to Pixabay Mediamodifier boxes businessman-2108029_1920</u>

<u>I am sure you could break up, flatten and put together as a screen Dividing Teams...</u>

<u>Perhaps this would help?</u>

*<u>**SO NOW IT IS NOW SCREEN DOWN TIME**</u>*

➢ <u>Here you need be re-introduced to Contract Bridge Bidding Rules in Game 3 before:- *↓</u>

➢ *The Four Suits are Ranked in the following order > (* The Highest to the Lowest).*

➢ *So we have * Spades>Hearts>Diamonds>Clubs.*

<u>Each Pair will be given a pack of 52 cards – the Host holds the two Jokers for later! THEN they must create the following 11 hands: 10 of 5 cards + the last one below of 2 cards, which must be a Pair! One point to make the designated hand plus bonus point for best hand. *</u>

<u>EXAMPLES BELOW</u>

1. Royal flush
A, K, Q, J, 10, all the same suit.

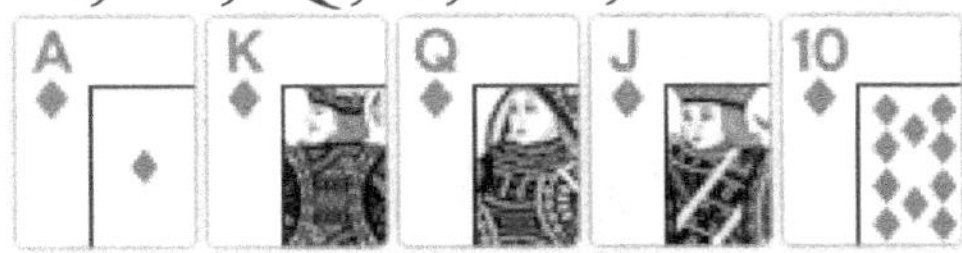 NB Bonus Point for top suit <u>*↑</u>

2. Straight flush
Five cards in a sequence, all in the same suit.

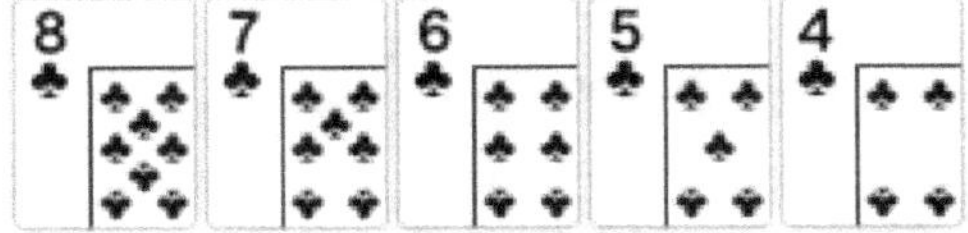 NB Bonus Point for top suit <u>*↑</u>

3. Four of a kind
All four cards of the same rank.

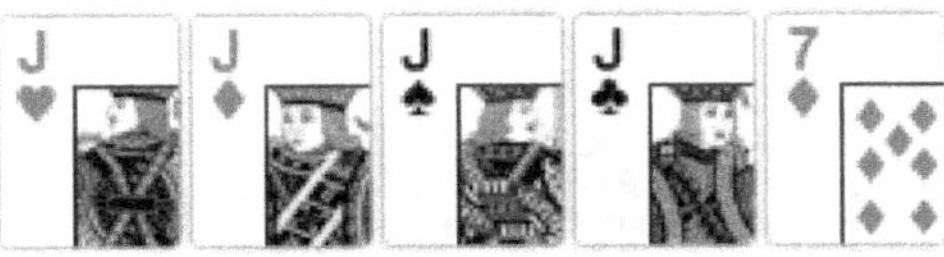 NB if the same ranking cards used – the 5th will determine Bonus Point <u>*↑</u>

4. Full house

Three of a kind with a pair.

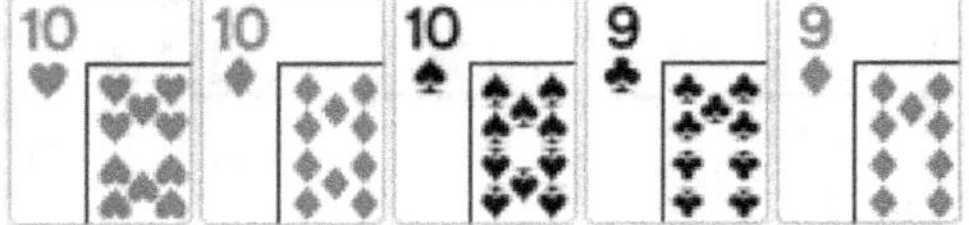 NB if the same 3 of a kind ranking cards used – then the pair will determine Bonus Point *↑

5. Flush

Any five cards of the same suit, but not in a sequence.

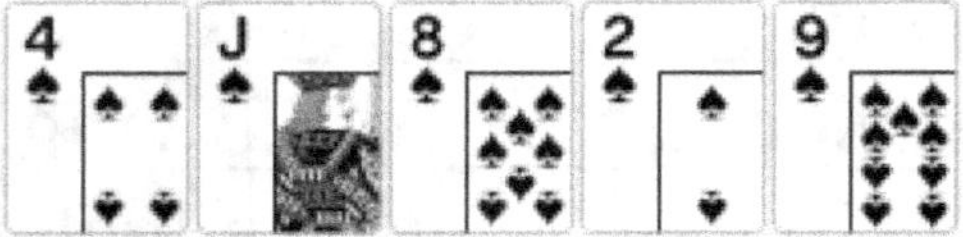 NB here the top ranking card will determine Bonus Point *↑ (If same then next high card and so on!

6. Straight

Five cards in a sequence, but not of the same suit.

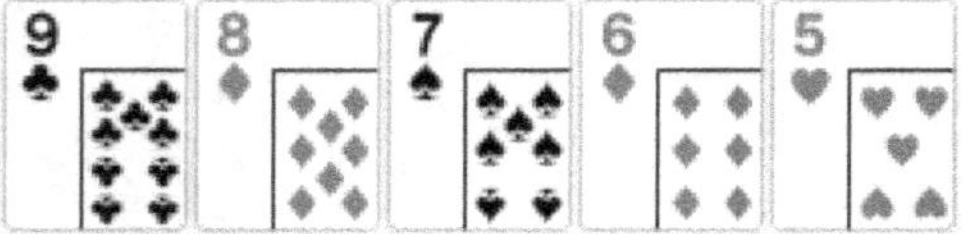 NB here the top ranking card will determine Bonus Point *↑

7. Three of a kind

Three cards of the same rank.

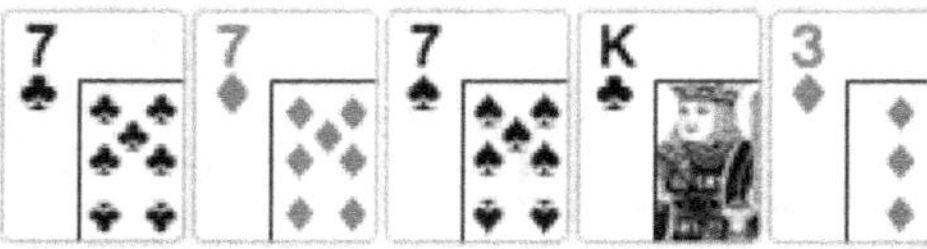 NB here if the same 3 of a kind, then the highest remaining card will determine Bonus Point *↑ (In example above that = the K of Clubs!

8. Two pair

Two different pairs.

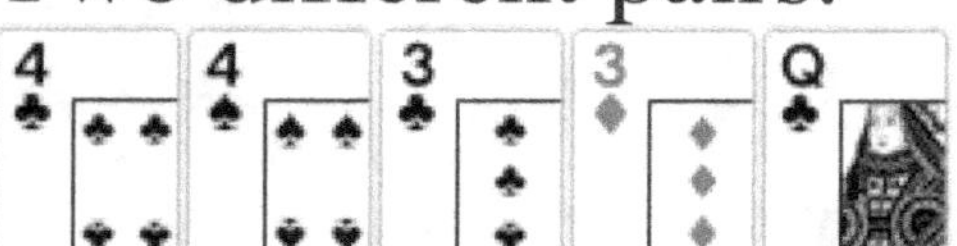 NB here the highest pair will determine Bonus Point *↑ (If same then the other highest pair! If identical then 5th card determines Bonus

9. Pair

Two cards of the same rank.
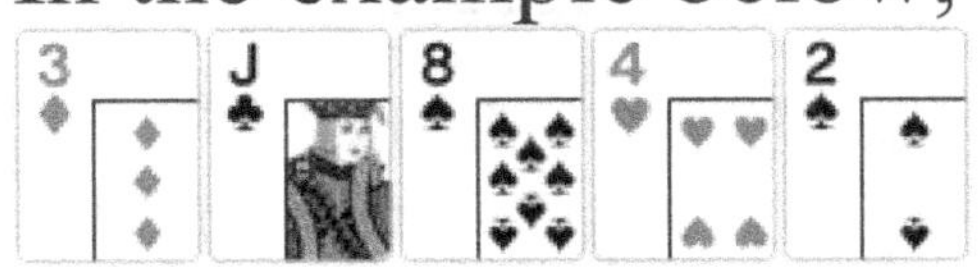 NB here the top pair will
determine Bonus Point *↑ (If same then next high card
and so on! The 8 is the next in line.

10. High Card

HIGH CARD ONLY – *no pairs etc*. NB here if
identical then next highest determines Bonus Point *↑
In the example below, the jack plays as the highest card.
The 8 is the next in line.

11. Another Pair
(As 9 Above)

a. **NB An Ace can be both low &/or high in a
straight, or in any flush.**

b. You must present your 11 Hands in Order above –
any not Correct will be classed as an **Invalid** Hand!

c. **INVALID** Hands will score **Minus One Point**!

d. Achieving Bonus Points explained above...   ↓

–

AFTER 10 MINUTES IT WILL BE <u>SCREEN UP TIME</u>

*When laid down cards are scored – **<u>do not remove them</u>**...
You will see when we go onto ...ANOTHER CARD GAME...*

>>>>>>>>>>>>

<u>New Partnerships Arranged.</u>
<u>Each Set # of Contestants will then be given their Two</u>
<u>Jokers, each count as any card nominated.</u>
<u>– From this you must re-create the first aforementioned</u>
<u>10 hands of 5 cards.</u>
<u>- Likely there will be some tactical joker held hand</u>
<u>changes.</u>
<u>The variable is the 11th Hand:-</u>

<u>the 4 cards must = 4 of a Kind!</u>

<u>Wait for The Screen# to come down AGAIN here!?</u>

THEN THE REARRANGING

TORMENT BEGINS AGAIN!

THEN ENJOY IT

IF IT DOESN'T

METAPHORICALLY

KILL YOU OFF FIRST!

So, it seems so far there has been an emphasis on the Adult side?

So, to address the balance we need venture back indoors where we can teach the kids a thing, or two, or more!?

Ignoring al that modern technological stuff and focus on games proper & historically found on dining room table homes:- there are literally a millennia!

But, and it is my literal Big But, my emphasis is on the educational and tactical arenas, where brain power can come to the fore, both in the descriptive verbal AND calculating mathematical i.e. for their brain development!

So, for me so many non-digital, can come to mind which have a home in various of my relative's households, in no particular order:-

1. Sevens – for those unfamiliar with this one:- is a shedding-type card game where the objective is to be the first player to get rid of all your cards by playing them onto a central layout. The game starts by dealing out a standard deck and begins with the seven of the first suit played, after which players add cards in sequential order, either ascending or descending, from the sevens already on the table. Players who cannot play a card must pass their turn.

2. Uno – another shedding game:- Played with a specially printed deck, the game is derived from the crazy eights family of card

games which, in turn, is based on the traditional German game of mau-mau.

3. Cluedo - known as Clue in North America, is a murder mystery game for three to six players (depending on editions) that was devised in 1943 by British board game designer Anthony E. Pratt. The object of the game is to determine who murdered the game's victim, where the crime took place, and which weapon was used.

4. Monopoly – Perhaps the most famous property board game in all its forms, from table to pocket size!

5. **Connect 4** – basically like noughts & crosses, but here you need to get 4 in row/line.

6. Downfall - where players strategically turn gears to race their tokens to the bottom.

7. Scrabble – again no introduction needed for this world famous word making game!

8. Heads Up – in its various forms, but basically for youngsters where who/what you are is stuck to your forehead (nowadays a live phone picture) and needs to be ascertained by word questions/clues.

9. Who am I? On the same lines as heads Up.

10. Ticket to Ride series, although more of an adult game of strategy/planning, which involves building railway routes across various regions (e.g., Europe or North America).

11.   Articulate, again perhaps a more adult type guessing game - a fast-talking, team-based board game where players describe as many words as possible to their teammates in 30 seconds.

12.   Trivial Pursuit, again more for the adults - a classic board game where players move around a board, answer trivia questions from different categories, and collect coloured wedges to win.

13.   And the hit & miss 'Chronology'- card game, by Buffalo Games, involves players guessing the correct chronological position of historical events to be the first to build a timeline of 10 cards.

But I shall just mention two specifically which are our regular standbys:- Quiddler & Rummikub.

The beauty of both is that it can be played by all ages, from aged Nanny to youngsters Jane & John!

18 RUMMIKUB/QUIDDLER – MATHS/SPELLING FUN

RUMMIKUB

Rummikub is a <u>tile-based game</u> for 2 to 4 players, combining elements of the card game <u>rummy</u> and <u>mah-jong</u>.

The first player to use all their tiles scores a positive score based on the total of the other players' hands, while the losers get negative scores.

An important feature of the game is that players can work with the tiles that have already been played by anyone.

The game can actually be played by more than 4 at once, if you wish to try, but, the simplest expedient is to have more than one set in the Family and so with 2 sets 8 can easily be accommodated, but make sure your tabletop can, too!

    A. *In addition to Adults, kids of a young age can play and should be encouraged to if only to develop their strategic and counting ability.*

    B. *Time limits are the area, which cause a certain grief, but they should be leniently exercised, within reason, as it is only a game.*

    C. *The main cause of time limit problems is that some, especially the older/more competitive try to calculate great combinations in their head and find that putting their thoughts into practice does not always work successfully.*

D. *And the upshot was/is that the board was/might be disorganised with tiles becoming out of place.*

E. *Thankfully, the modern I-Phone has in-built a camera system and (we all know those most likely to try the impossible, so to speak) all we need do is take a snap shot before they take their turn.*

F. *Two things of special note before you play with others: it is usually the playing of Jokers. The earliest editions rules covering Joker moves differ from the later, easier editions, so ensure you know which you are playing, in addition to any other local variations.*

G. *All you need now is to work out the Sweet Prizes!*

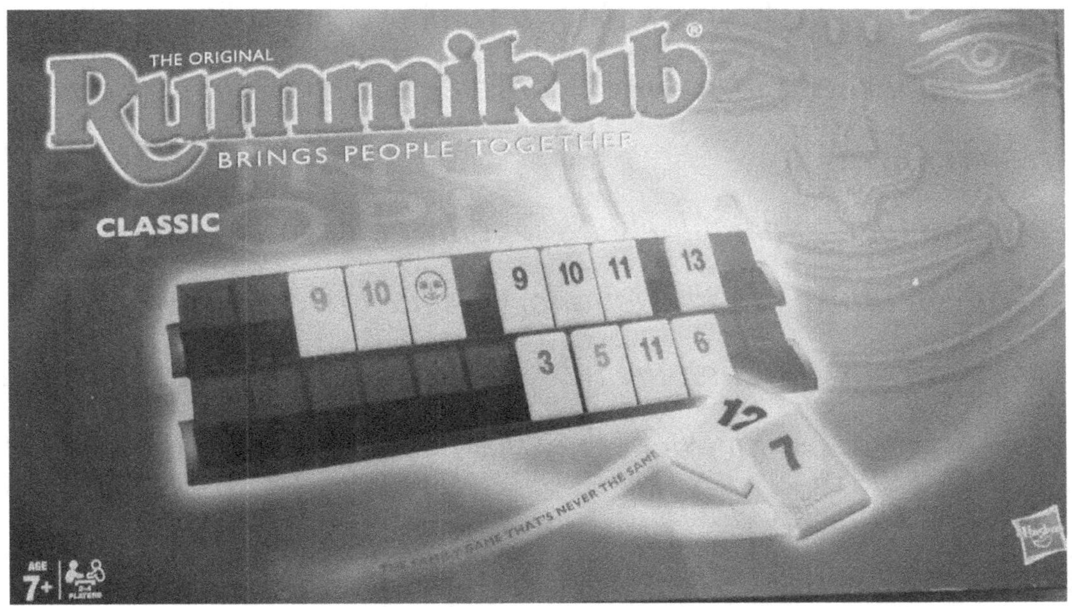

OFF YOU GO TRY ME

<u>QUIDDLER</u>

Quiddler is in the main a word game.

Players compete by spelling acceptable English words from cards in hands of increasing size, each card worth various points.

The person with the highest total after the agreed number of rounds is the winner.

As you get more tiles to play with you might notice a slight resemblance to Gin Rummy, not unlike Rummikub above.

A. *The beauty of the game is that up to 8 can play at once.*

B. *In addition to Adults, kids of a young age can play and should be encouraged to, if only to develop their vocabulary and counting ability.*

C. *To aid them particularly I adapt the rules to introduce the Universal use of the Dictionary: Whilst person 1 is trying to lay him/herself out, then the next to play, person 2, can search for words to assist him/her; they pass the Dictionary on when it is their turn to lay down.*

D. *The Dictionary use works well and the only dissenter would be the person who starts and so would be the last to get a turn!*

E. *Additionally, it is best to keep your 'accepted' dictionary with the game to avoid problems in the future.*

F. It should be borne in mind this is not Scrabble with its obscure word use and so we can dispense with their overlong accepted 2 letter words chart. Only what is in your Dictionary, within the Rules, are acceptable! These will be well known through playing practice!

G. Time limits are the area, which cause a certain grief, but they should be leniently exercised, within reason, as it is only a game.

H. Similarly, the 'Challenge' system, where the user should be given another reasonably timed try.

I. All you need now is to work out the Sweet Prizes!

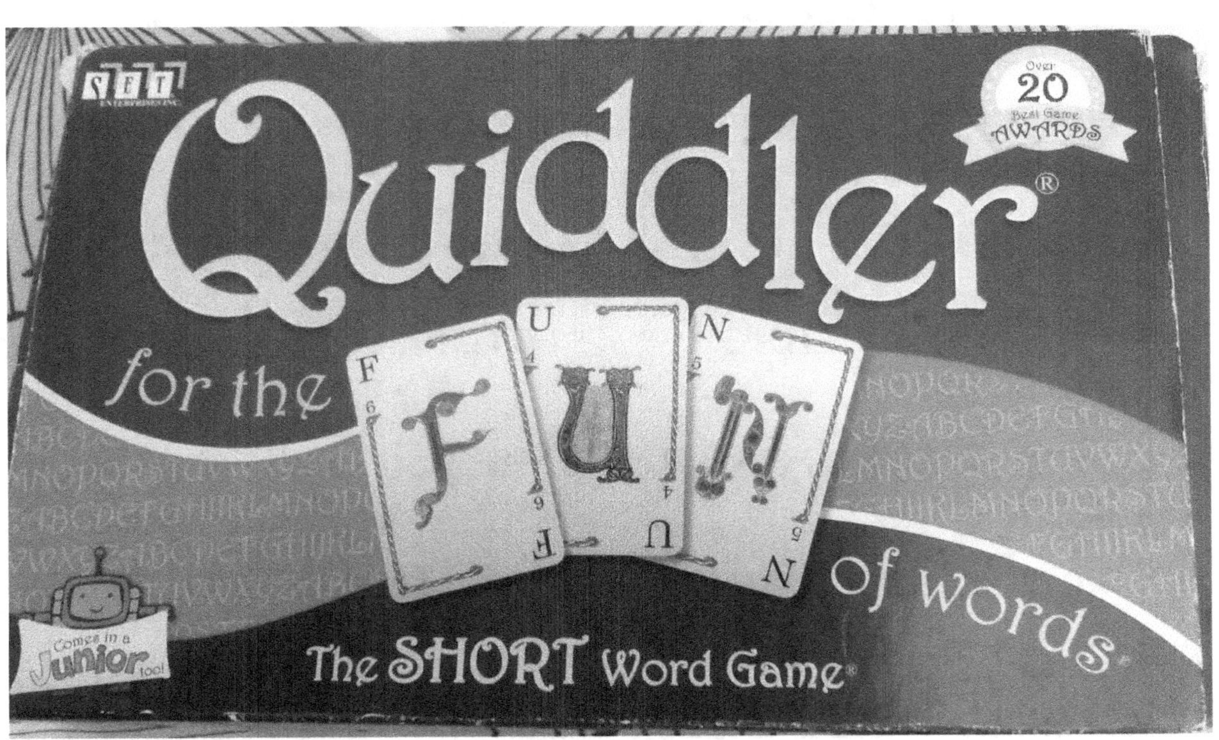

<u>AND JUST ONE MORE CARD GAME</u>
<u>WHERE LOSING IS WINNING!?</u>

19 KIRKE – THE CARD GAME YOU WIN BY LOSING!
THIS HAS BEEN IN MY FAMILY
FOR GENERATIONS...
SO HERE WE ARE, INDOORS, OR OUT: WE CAN PLAY

WITH COUNTERS/SWEETS, OR EVEN MONEY.

BUT, AND IT IS A VERY BIG LOSING BUT,

10p PER POINT IS A REASONABLE FAMILY STAKE.

IF THE OLDER KIDS PLAY

AND LIKELY THEY WOULD WANT TO, TOO,

IF SWEETS WERE THE REWARD FOR WINNING >>>

SAY 10 FOR THE HIGHEST RANKING AND LESS AS WE

GO DOWN THE 2nd/3rd/4th ETC. PLACE SCALE,

DEPENDING ON THE NUMBERS PLAYING#↓

(PS For those against their kids getting addicted we need tell them the game is purely education e.g. learning how to count; experiencing the good with the bad i.e. learning how to lose as well as winning; and most importantly it brings out the important human interaction need that to satisfy that gregarious experience/need in us all!)

A11=KIRKE (KING/QUEEN)
SCORING PERMUTATIONS

LOSING POINTS	3 PLAY	4 PLAY	5 PLAY	6 PLAY	7 PLAY	8 PLAY	9 PLAY	SPECIAL NOTES
NO JACKS 4 x 20	80	80	80	80	80	80	80	# See 'Play without' instructions and 'number of tricks' below for differ player numbers #
NO QUEENS 4 x 20	80	80	80	80	80	80	80	
NO TRICKS # x #	136	130	120	120	119	120	100	
NO HEARTS # x 10	130	130	130	120	130	120	120	
NO King of Hearts 1 x # xxx	54	70	60	50	51	50	40	
NO LAST 2 Tricks 2 x 15	30	30	30	30	30	30	30	
ALL IN	510	520	500	480	490	480	450	
*TOTAL	1020	1040	1000	960	980	960	900	

AND NOW
THE GAME GOES
ON ITS POINTS HEAD

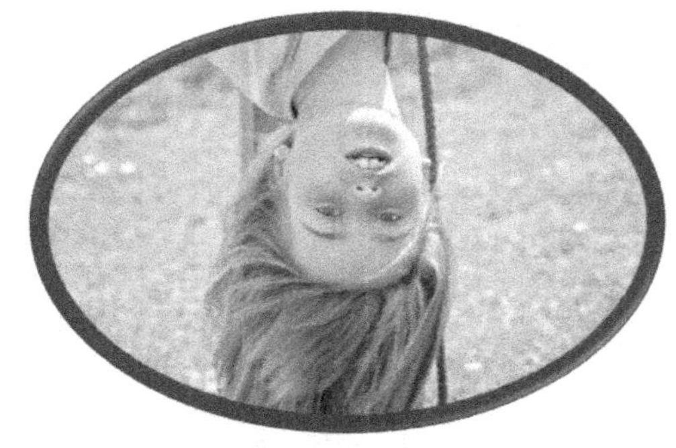

And so, From P19 We welcome our own upside down card girl! **(From losing the least points to winning the most!)**

WINNING POINTS	EACH PLAYER HAS ONE ROUND OF CHOOSING TRUMPS							PLAY WITH OUT:
3 PLAYERS = 3 rounds								2 OF CLUBS
each trick 20 points								
17 tricks x 3 TOTAL	1020							
4 PLAYERS = 4 rounds								NONE
each trick 20 points								
13 tricks x 4 TOTAL		1040						
5 PLAYERS = 5 rounds								BLACK 2s
each trick 20 points								
10 tricks x 5 TOTAL			1000					
6 PLAYERS = 6 rounds								ALL THE 2s
each trick 20 points								
8 tricks x 6 TOTAL				960				
7 PLAYERS = 7 rounds								2 of clubs, spades & diamonds
each trick 20 points								
7 tricks x 7 TOTAL					980			
8 PLAYERS = 8 rounds								ALL THE 2s
each trick 20 points								
6 rounds x 8 TOTAL						960		
9 PLAYERS = 9 rounds								ALL THE 2s plus 3 of clubs, diamonds & spades.
each trick 20 points								
5 rounds x 9 TOTAL							900	

Not ideal for 3, or 9.   #↑   **Best is 4/5/6/7/8.**

For the losing rounds the amount per trick and the King of Hearts differ from each other to balance the scores i.e. For 3 = 17 tricks @ 8 points; for 4 = 13 tricks @ 10; for 5 = 10 tricks @ 12; for 6 = 8 tricks @ 15; for 7 = 7 tricks @ 17; for 8 = 6 tricks @ 20; for 9 = 5 tricks @ 20.   *

The deal is passed around to the left after each round; the person to the dealer's left always leads; the dealer picks trumps during the winning points rounds.

During *'Winning Points'* rounds one must always follow suit, but when not having the suit led then one can trump or discard.

During *'Losing Points'* rounds one must always follow suit, but, when not having the suit led, then this is the time to dump your opponent with one of your loss attracting cards like Jacks, Queens & especially-immediately - the King of Hearts, when his turn comes around [xxx]!

During *'No Hearts, No King of Hearts, All In'* rounds Hearts cannot be led until you have only that suit left in your hand.

IF PLAYING FOR MONEY YOU SHOULD FIND
THAT AT THE END OF THE GAME
THE MINUS SCORE TOTALS
ALWAYS =
THE PLUS SCORE TOTALS
SO THE LOSERS PAY THE WINNERS
IF NOT THEN THE SCORER HAS MADE A MISTAKE

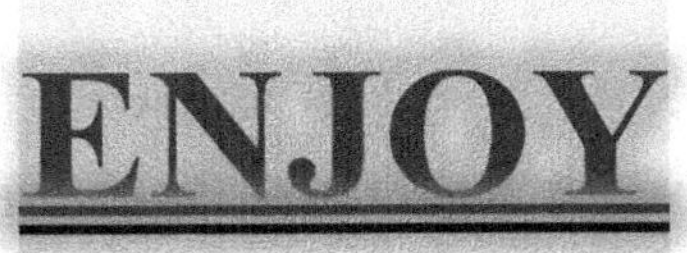

ENJOY

(IT GETS EASIER THE MORE TIMES YOU PLAY!

Now comes Senior Adult Christmas Winding Down Time.

I suppose after all that eating/drinking you'd think you should burn off so many of the kids' calories and rid them of the hyper-active sugar content, but, and it is that usual Big But, it applies both ways and would you really like to exert yourself when there is a more relaxed alternative and guaranteed to keep the (grand) children + friend(s) quiet AND focused?

> *Although, you can use this ploy at any time when*
> *IT all becomes too much like hard work!?*

AND there are always those times Mummy wants Daddy & kids to leave her alone in peace to get on with things!

And so we have my variety on the Treasure Hunt Game and all you'll need is

a) a pencil and pad with a few sheets attached for each child

b) that each child taking part can write letters and numbers without great assistance!

1. First the Bribe
2. Say there will be prizes
3. But add they will be hidden (not really – see below) *
4. And clues to their whereabouts will only materialize afterwards
5. After what?

- This will take the form of a (Leisurely for you) Walk around the block.
- Before you set off ensure each child has their name on their sheets.

And off you all go: the object being that the children write down Car Registration Numbers of Stationary Vehicles they see without crossing the road with their chosen letter *** within it.

And yes they can look, _but not enter_ people's gardens!

Silly, you might say, because they'll each end up with pad full of a multiplicity of number plate numbers?

Well, here comes the twist – and here it pays to know your Local Code – So, if in London you avoid giving a child an 'L' and never allocate an 'O' as it will get confused with Zero! Similarly, avoid the vowels which could greatly inflate the numbers collected.

If you look up the DLVA website you'll know what not to include in your area – oddly enough 'B', 'R', 'T', are good random choices! ***

So, before you set off you ask the children which of the letters you have set before them they wish to select. ***

And off you go.

As off they go collecting!

And if their selected letter appears on a number plate they write the whole registration on their pad. You might also find on occasion that the same number plate applies to two children at one time.

Because of the nature of this game being fraught with delay as the kids slowly/diligently hunt/find/list number plate numbers, you'll find the pace is naturally sedate – great for grannies & grandads!

All you need take care of is the encroachment onto the road – but you'd do that naturally whenever out with the kids, don't you?

There again keep to the local minor roads!

When you get home separate the children & get them each, with their lists hidden from the rest, to itemise how many of number 1s, 2s, 3s, etc up to 9s, they got.

Then from a pack of cards extract an ace, a 2, a 3, a 4, a 5, a 6, a 7,

a 8, lastly a 9.

Shuffle them, then lay them face down on the floor. *

Ask one child to point to the card you should first pick up – show it. *

If it is a 3, then the child who had the most 3s collected gets to pick a wrapped sweet prize from say the sack in your possession. *

The same person gets to pick the next card.

And so on.

If one child has got his second prize he/she drops out **.

Stipulations:- say you have 4 children playing, then the maximum number of prizes s/b 6 – so two children can have a max of 2 prizes each **, whilst the other two children are guaranteed at least one each e.g. once the 5th prize is won, the remaining one is given to the child who has won none.

However, if at the 5th prize stage onlyone has won 2, then obviously they are out and only the remaining 3 will vie for that second prize!

So there you have the best of 3 relaxing worlds:

1. A leisurely walk around the block +
2. A leisurely sitting about whilst the kids list their numbers
3. A further leisurely sitting about whilst the kids eat the goodies

ENJOY

WELL I HOPE YOU ENJOYED MY GAMES DIVERSION EXCURSIONS

AND SO IT IS BACK TO CAKE BASICS >>>>

21 CHRISTMAS > MYA'S CAKE (Part 2 of 2) COVERING

THAT CHRISTMAS CAKE REVISIT AT ITS POST BAKE AND POST SETTLEMENT STAGE

<u>**POST BAKE**</u>

- After baking take out of the oven to cool.

- If your baking tin has tightening clip on its side – open this out and remove.

- But, I do not remove the cake from its base; all this I place on say a wooden chopping board, until no longer warm..

- Nor do I remove any surrounding baking/greaseproof paper!

- When happy the cake is no longer warm cover/fold-in the outer layer of greaseproof paper and then cover with more if any gaps;

- Then enclose from bottom to top in foil, making the cake virtually airtight and set aside for a month or so;

- <u>Do not place foil in direct contact with the cake as it will stick & may rust?</u>

- <u>*Open up periodically (your personal alcohol content choice)* [xx] *to use up the left over liquor saved above (And more some?)* [xx]</u>

- *Here skewer prick the cake so it will easily absorb liquor.*

- *Then recover with greaseproof paper, then reseal with the foil.*

THAT CHRISTMAS CAKE REVISIT AT ITS POST BAKE AND POST SETTLEMENT STAGE
POST SETTLEMENT STAGE

> Firstly remove all the greaseproof paper & foil; then remove the metal tin base, which should be retained as a template for the size of marzipan/icing to cover the cake top, #

A week before possibly eating decorate with marzipan and leave a day, or two, for it to set, then add the icing & finally with leftover roasted almonds (* if you wish add left over marzipan (in balls), or separately, coat them with hot chocolate!*

Then you would need-

a. 2 slabs of ready-made marzipan, even try the brandy flavoured

b. 2 packets at least of ordinary icing, or preferably fondant, ready to roll out like the marzipan.

c. But not for me Royal Icing as it gets too hard and sharp, especially with pointy ends!

d. Seedless jam to put around the cake to attract the marzipan;

e. I prefer raspberry &/or apricot preserve!

f. Remember [1] only **coat the cake outer with jam AFTER** you have successfully rolled out the marzipan to wholly fit all round!

g. Remember [2] when rolling out the marzipan slabs and fondant icing slabs, which I prefer, you need ***periodically*** sprinkle this work surface with icing sugar to stop the icing/marzipan sticking to everything!

h. Roll out as thinly as you dare but sufficient to cut to fit #, just as you did with the base of the tin and the fitting greaseproof paper

i. Getting the marzipan sides sorted will be more of a challenge!

j. After the icing, roast another almonds batch to decorate top.

k. ↑ (**a <> j**) *above will be two other separate stages you can involve your greedy little nibblers where the jam and leftover marzipan and icing sugar will be their sweet targets - again if they agree to wash/dry/clear up afterwards!*

Remember [3] *care with icing sugar*
*<> add the water **sparingly** to the icing <> not vice-versa!*

This book is dedicated to John's memory and a certain famous *Natasha*, too, whom he met & always had the kids foremost in her *Muddy Puddles Countryphile* Mind!
But, now, too, like John, *a Distant Memory*!

Anyhow, back to the *present* and I hope you think this of my *present* to you, so those words,

- *"Mummy/Daddy come and play with me/us!"*

DO NOT
fill you full of,
"*Later Dear!*"
***Defensive Dread*!!!**
But, more of
Gleeful Fun Sharing Anticipation!

(Well, at least I haven't left you short of ideas!)

Regards from the Copyright Writing Battle Front
Banish Anguish Michael
AND Family

AND FOR THE BIG CHRISTMAS/BOXING DAY/NEW YEAR

WHO-DUNNIT READ MY >>>

WHO STOLE OUR CHRISTMAS PRESENTS?
SCREAMED SETH & JUDE!:
V3 = THE THREE DAY HEISTS

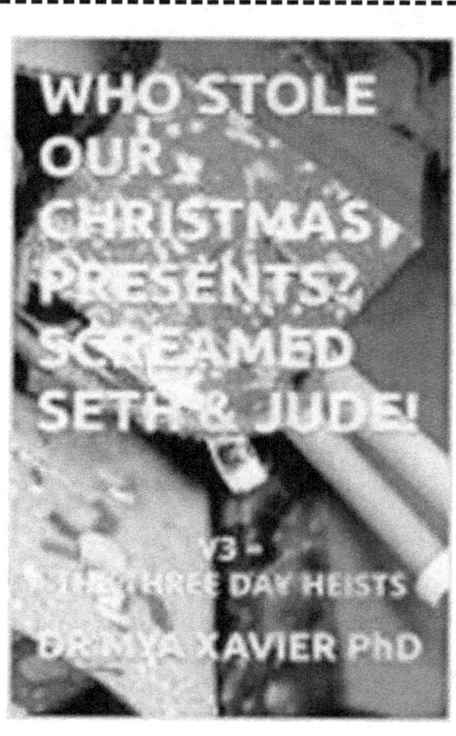

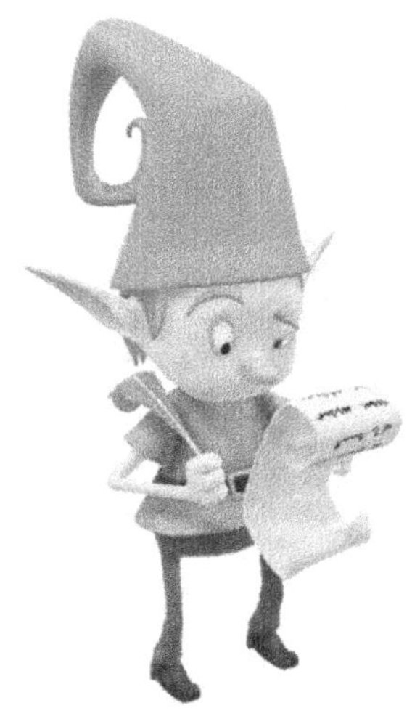

MR ELF HELPER

SEES AND KNOWS

MORE THAN YOU THINK

AT CHRISTMAS!

REGARDS Dr Mya Xavier PhD

>>>